Review of the DoD-GEIS Influenza Programs

Strengthening Global Surveillance and Response

Committee for the Assessment of DoD-GEIS Influenza Surveillance and Response Programs

Board on Global Health

INSTITUTE OF MEDICINE
OF THE NATIONAL ACADEMIES

THE NATIONAL ACADEMIES PRESS
Washington, D.C.
www.nap.edu

THE NATIONAL ACADEMIES PRESS 500 Fifth Street, N.W. Washington, DC 20001

NOTICE: The project that is the subject of this report was approved by the Governing Board of the National Research Council, whose members are drawn from the councils of the National Academy of Sciences, the National Academy of Engineering, and the Institute of Medicine. The members of the committee responsible for the report were chosen for their special competences and with regard for appropriate balance.

This study was supported by Contract No. W81XWH-06-C-0381 (DoD-7741) between the National Academy of Sciences and the Department of Defense. Any opinions, findings, conclusions, or recommendations expressed in this publication are those of the author(s) and do not necessarily reflect the view of the organizations or agencies that provided support for this project.

International Standard Book Number-13: 978-0-309-11010-5
International Standard Book Number-10: 0-309-11010-6

Additional copies of this report are available from the National Academies Press, 500 Fifth Street, N.W., Lockbox 285, Washington, DC 20055; (800) 624-6242 or (202) 334-3313 (in the Washington metropolitan area); Internet, http://www.nap.edu.

For more information about the Institute of Medicine, visit the IOM home page at: **www.iom.edu.**

Printed in the United States of America.

The serpent has been a symbol of long life, healing, and knowledge among almost all cultures and religions since the beginning of recorded history. The serpent adopted as a logotype by the Institute of Medicine is a relief carving from ancient Greece, now held by the Staatliche Museen in Berlin.

Suggested citation: Institute of Medicine (IOM). 2008. *Review of the DOD-GEIS influenza programs: Strengthening global surveillance and response.* Washington, DC: The National Academies Press.

"Knowing is not enough; we must apply.
Willing is not enough; we must do."
—Goethe

INSTITUTE OF MEDICINE
OF THE NATIONAL ACADEMIES

Advising the Nation. Improving Health.

THE NATIONAL ACADEMIES

Advisers to the Nation on Science, Engineering, and Medicine

The **National Academy of Sciences** is a private, nonprofit, self-perpetuating society of distinguished scholars engaged in scientific and engineering research, dedicated to the furtherance of science and technology and to their use for the general welfare. Upon the authority of the charter granted to it by the Congress in 1863, the Academy has a mandate that requires it to advise the federal government on scientific and technical matters. Dr. Ralph J. Cicerone is president of the National Academy of Sciences.

The **National Academy of Engineering** was established in 1964, under the charter of the National Academy of Sciences, as a parallel organization of outstanding engineers. It is autonomous in its administration and in the selection of its members, sharing with the National Academy of Sciences the responsibility for advising the federal government. The National Academy of Engineering also sponsors engineering programs aimed at meeting national needs, encourages education and research, and recognizes the superior achievements of engineers. Dr. Charles M. Vest is president of the National Academy of Engineering.

The **Institute of Medicine** was established in 1970 by the National Academy of Sciences to secure the services of eminent members of appropriate professions in the examination of policy matters pertaining to the health of the public. The Institute acts under the responsibility given to the National Academy of Sciences by its congressional charter to be an adviser to the federal government and, upon its own initiative, to identify issues of medical care, research, and education. Dr. Harvey V. Fineberg is president of the Institute of Medicine.

The **National Research Council** was organized by the National Academy of Sciences in 1916 to associate the broad community of science and technology with the Academy's purposes of furthering knowledge and advising the federal government. Functioning in accordance with general policies determined by the Academy, the Council has become the principal operating agency of both the National Academy of Sciences and the National Academy of Engineering in providing services to the government, the public, and the scientific and engineering communities. The Council is administered jointly by both Academies and the Institute of Medicine. Dr. Ralph J. Cicerone and Dr. Charles M. Vest are chair and vice chair, respectively, of the National Research Council.

www.national-academies.org

COMMITTEE FOR THE ASSESSMENT OF DOD-GEIS INFLUENZA SURVEILLANCE AND RESPONSE PROGRAMS

MYRON M. LEVINE, M.D., D.T.P.H. (*Chair*), Professor and Director, Simon and Bessie Grollman Distinguished Professor, Center for Vaccine Development, University of Maryland School of Medicine

CAROL CARDONA, D.V.M., Ph.D., Associate Veterinarian, Associate Specialist in Cooperative Extension, Veterinary Medicine Extension, University of California, Davis

WALTER DOWDLE, Ph.D., The Task Force for Child Survival and Development

TIMOTHY GERMANN, Ph.D., Technical Staff Member, Applied Science & Methods Development Group, Los Alamos National Laboratory

MARY GILCHRIST, Ph.D., Director, Bureau of Laboratory Sciences, State Laboratory Institute, Department of Public Health, The Commonwealth of Massachusetts

JAMES M. HUGHES, M.D., Director, Program in Global Infectious Disease, Center for Global Safe Water, School of Medicine and Rollins School of Public Health, Emory University

K. MILLS McNEILL, Ph.D., M.D., Director, Public Health Laboratory, Mississippi State Department of Health

PETER PALESE, Ph.D., Professor and Chair Department of Microbiology, Mount Sinai School of Medicine

KENNEDY FRANCIS SHORTRIDGE, Ph.D., D.Sc., Emeritus Professor, The University of Hong Kong and Honorary Professor, Department of Micobiology, The University of Hong Kong, Hong Kong SAR, China, Honorary Professor, Department of Molecular Medicine and Pathology, The University of Auckland, Auckland, New Zealand

JAMES TIBENDERANA, M.B.CH.B., M.Phil., Ph.D., Drug Policy Change Specialist/Epidemiologist Malaria Consortium, Uganda

Board Liaison

PHILIP K. RUSSELL, M.D., (*Board on Global Health Liaison*) Former Director, Office of Research and Development Coordination, Office of the Assistant Secretary for Public Health Emergency Preparedness, U.S. Department of Health and Human Services

Project Staff

PATRICK W. KELLEY, M.D., Dr.P.H., Director, Boards on Global Health and African Science Academy Development

RICK ERDTMANN, M.D., M.P.H., Director, Boards on Military and Veterans Health and Medical Follow-up Agency

J. ALICE NIXON, M.A., Study Director

KIMBERLY WEINGARTEN, Research Assistant

ANGELA MENSAH, Senior Program Assistant (November 2006–April 2007)

EMILY S. MEYER, Intern (February 2007–May 2007)

Reviewers

This report has been reviewed in draft form by individuals chosen for their diverse perspectives and technical expertise, in accordance with procedures approved by the NRC's Report Review Committee. The purpose of this independent review is to provide candid and critical comments that will assist the institution in making its published report as sound as possible and to ensure that the report meets institutional standards for objectivity, evidence, and responsiveness to the study charge. The review comments and draft manuscript remain confidential to protect the integrity of the deliberative process. We wish to thank the following individuals for their review of this report:

Donald S. Burke, Graduate School of Public Health, University of Pittsburgh
Philip E. Coyle III, Science Strategies, LLC
Kathy Edwards, Division of Pediatric Infectious Diseases, Department of Pediatrics, Vanderbilt University School of Medicine
Benson Estambale, College of Health Sciences, University of Nairobi Institute of Tropical and Infectious Diseases,
Alison P. Galvani, Division of Epidemiology of Microbial Diseases, Yale University School of Medicine
Kathleen F. Gensheimer, Medical Epidemiology Section, Division of Infectious Diseases, Maine Department of Health and Human Service
Lance Jennings, Canterbury Heath Laboratories, Christchurch, New Zealand

Daniel Lavanchy, Epidemic and Pandemic Alert and Response, Office for Alert and Response Operations, World Health Organization
Graeme Laver, Australian National University, Professor Emeritus
Mark Miller, Fogarty International Center, National Institutes of Health
Frederick A. Murphy, Galveston Department of Pathology, University of Texas Medical Branch
Douglas M. Watts, Department of Pathology, Center for Biodefense and Emerging Infectious Diseases, University of Texas Medical Branch

Although the reviewers listed above have provided many constructive comments and suggestions, they were not asked to endorse the conclusions or recommendations nor did they see the final draft of the report before its release. The review of this report was overseen by **Dr. David R. Challoner,** Vice President for Health Affairs, Emeritus, University of Florida, and **Charles C.J. Carpenter,** the Miriam Hospital and Brown University. Appointed by the National Research Council and Institute of Medicine, they were responsible for making certain that an independent examination of this report was carried out in accordance with institutional procedures and that all review comments were carefully considered. Responsibility for the final content of this report rests entirely with the authoring committee and the institution.

Preface

Influenza in humans is an acute respiratory disease caused by RNA viruses that continually undergo genetic change, allowing seasonal epidemics as the viruses evolve in subtle ways that permit them to evade preexisting immunity in portions of the human population. During seasonal epidemics, the very young and the elderly bear the brunt of mortality from influenza. However, every few decades a fundamental antigenic shift occurs in the virus, resulting in the emergence of a strikingly new influenza viral strain to which most of the human population is susceptible. If the new virus is particularly virulent, as well as antigenically distinct and readily transmissible between humans, a pandemic can ensue that represents a public health emergency with likely severe human and economic repercussions. The two most recent pandemics (1957 and 1968) are known to have resulted from a human influenza virus acquiring genes from an avian virus, resulting in a "reassorted" virus.

Three pandemics caused by influenza A viruses occurred in the 20th century, including 1918-1919 (H1N1 virus), 1957 (H2N2 virus), and 1968 (H3N2 virus). Among these, the 1918-1919 pandemic stands out because of the particularly severe clinical disease observed and the unusual epidemiologic behavior that ensued in which healthy young adults, in addition to the very young and elderly, suffered high mortality. During the 1918-1919 pandemic, U.S. armed services personnel on military installations in the United States experienced unprecedented fatality rates.

Fundamental strategies to minimize the impact of the next pandemic include the maintenance of a global surveillance system to detect emerging shifted influenza viruses, the rapid development of vaccines based on the newly emerged "shifted" strains, and use of stockpiled antiviral drugs. As both the 1957 and 1968 pandemic viruses apparently originated in East Asia, a critical component of current global influenza surveillance is based on the early detection of influenza-like disease and collection of influenza viruses from Asia.

In 1997 an outbreak of influenza in chickens in Hong Kong due to a highly lethal H5N1 avian influenza A virus also caused 18 human cases, of which six were fatal. Since 2004, other avian H5N1 viruses have wreaked havoc among domestic poultry in East and Southeast Asia and have also caused more than 300 human cases (among close human contacts of poultry), of which 60 percent were fatal. Thus far H5N1 viruses have not attained the capacity to transmit readily from human to human but the United States must be vigilant.

In 1996, the Executive Office of the President of the United States issued a Presidential Decision Directive declaring that national and international capabilities for infectious disease surveillance, prevention, and response were insufficient to protect the health of U.S. citizens from emerging infectious diseases and called on U.S. federal agencies to remedy the situation. The Department of Defense (DoD) Global Emerging Infections Surveillance and Response System (GEIS), established in 1997, represents the DoD's response to that Presidential Decision Directive. GEIS's focus is primarily on sentinel surveillance of indigenous and expatriate populations for certain infectious disease targets, including influenza. For many decades the DoD has maintained a series of overseas medical research facilities in Asia, Africa, and Latin America that have been well poised to participate in the detection of emerging infectious disease threats. Collectively, these DoD facilities constitute an extraordinary array of surveillance assets.

In 2006, through the National Defense Authorization Act, Congress provided a $39 million supplement to GEIS, specifically to expand surveillance and response capabilities with respect to the threat of pandemic influenza of avian virus origin. An IOM Committee was assembled at the request of the DoD to evaluate how the GEIS pandemic influenza surveillance and response program utilized the supplemental funds, strengthened influenza surveillance efforts domestically and internationally, integrated DoD efforts with those of other Federal agencies, coordinated activities with host countries (and neighboring countries in regional efforts), and collaborated with the World Health Organization and other international agencies engaged in influenza pandemic preparedness. Toward this end, a Committee was assembled with expertise in influenza, epidemiology, public health laboratory management, virology, veterinary and human medicine, global health and military preventive medicine. The Committee made site visits to the DoD overseas medical research units where GEIS-supported projects are under way, as well as to key military medical laboratories within the United States involved in influenza surveillance. The findings of the Committee are summarized in this report, along with a series of recommendations.

The Committee found that the DoD's overseas medical research units constitute an impressive network that has laudably utilized the supplemental funding to strengthen influenza surveillance, in addition to continuing their historically primary research activities. Perhaps the Committee's most overarching recommendation is that DoD-GEIS headquarters should be formally charged with providing overall managerial and technical oversight (quality assurance, safety, etc.) and interagency communication for the multi-service influenza and respiratory disease surveillance program and the revised coordination structure. Part of this should be a codified chain of accountability to include timely reporting of findings. If the full set of recommendations are acted upon, the Committee is confident that the DoD-GEIS's key role in global surveillance will be further strengthened and its effectiveness enhanced.

Myron M. Levine, M.D., D.T.P.H.
Chair

Contents

LIST OF FIGURES

LIST OF TABLES

LIST OF BOXES

Abbreviations and Acronyms

AAALAC	American Association for the Accreditation of Laboratory Animal Care
AFCOM	U.S. African Command
AFIOH	Air Force Institute for Operational Health
AFIP	Armed Forces Institute of Pathology
AFMIC	Armed Forces Medical Intelligence Center
AFRIMS	Armed Forces Research Institute of Medical Sciences, Thailand
AFRO	WHO Regional Office for Africa
AI	avian influenza
AI/PI	avian influenza/pandemic influenza
AI/PI EPP	Avian Influenza/Pandemic Influenza Emergency Preparedness Plan
AMSA	U.S. Army's medical surveillance activity
ARI	acute respiratory infection
ASD-HA	Assistant Secretary of Defense for Health Affairs
BSL-2	biosafety level 2
BSL-3	biosafety level 3
BSL-3E	biosafety level 3 enhanced
BUMED	Naval Bureau of Medicine and Surgery
CDC	Centers for Disease Control and Prevention
CDHAM	Center for Disaster and Humanitarian Assistance
CENTCOM	U.S. Central Command

CHPPM	U.S. Army Center for Health Promotion and Preventive Medicine
COCOM	Combatant Command
CONOPS	concept of operations
CONUS	continental U.S.
CPE	cytopathic effect
DCM	Deputy Chief of Mission
DGE	Directorate of General Epidemiology
DHP	Defense Health Program
DHS	U.S. Department of Homeland Security
DoD	U.S. Department of Defense
DoS	U.S. Department of State
DSO	Defense Science Organization
EDCD	Epidemiology and Disease Control Division
EID	emerging infectious disease
EMRO	Eastern Mediterranean Regional Office
EUCOM	U.S. European Command
EWORS	Early Warning Outbreak Recognition System
FAO	Food and Agricultural Organization
FDA	Food and Drug Administration
FISC	Fleet and Industrial Supply Center
FRI	febrile respiratory illness
FSN	foreign service nationals
FTE	full-time equivalent
GAINS	Global Avian Influenza Network Surveillance
GEIS	Global Emerging Infections and Surveillance Response System
GLP	good laboratory practice
GOARN	Global Outbreak Alert Response Network
GTZ	German Agency for Technical Cooperation
HA	hemagglutinin
HAI	human avian influenza
HHS	U.S. Department for Health and Human Services
HIV	human immunodeficiency virus
HJF	Henry M. Jackson Foundation
HPAI	highly pathogenic avian influenza
ICEID	International Conference on Emerging Infectious Diseases
IDSA	Infectious Diseases Society of America
IEC	information, education, and communication
IEIP	International Emerging Infections Program
IF	immunofluorescence
ILI	influenza-like illness

INS	Instituto Nacional de Salud Peru
IOM	Institute of Medicine
IRB	institutional review board
ITI	Idaho Technology Incorporated
JHU/APL	Johns Hopkins University Applied Physics Laboratory
JISWG	Joint Influenza Surveillance Working Group
KEMRI	Kenya Medical Research Institute
LANL	Los Alamos National Laboratory
LES	locally employed staff
LRN	Laboratory Response Network
MAAIF	Ministry of Agriculture, Animal Industry, and Fisheries
MDCK	Madin-Darby canine kidney
MHS	military health system
MIDRP	Military Infectious Diseases Research Program
MoA	Ministry of Agriculture
MoE	Ministry of Environment
MoH	Ministry of Health
MoHP	Ministry of Health and Population
MoPH	Ministry of Public Health
MoU	memorandum of understanding
MTF	Medical Treatment Facilities
MUWRP	Makerere University Walter Reed Project
NAMRID	Naval Medical Research Institute Detachment
NAMRU-2	Naval Medical Research Unit No. 2, Indonesia
NAMRU-3	Naval Medical Research Unit No. 3, Egypt
NASA	National Aeronautics and Space Administration
NBIC	National Biosurveillance Integration Center
NCD	Newcastle disease
NCLE	National Center for Laboratory and Epidemiology
NEHC	Navy Environmental Health Center
NGO	nongovernmental organization
NHRC	Naval Health Research Center, San Diego, CA
NIC	National Influenza Center
NIH	National Institutes of Health
NMRC	Naval Medical Research Center
NMRCD	Naval Medical Research Center Detachment, Peru
NORTHCOM	U.S. Northern Command
NPHL	National Public Health Laboratory
NRDL	National Respiratory Disease Laboratory
NSTC-7	National Science and Technology Council, Executive Office of the President, Presidential Decision Directive
NTF	National Task Force

OASDHA	Office of the Assistant Secretary of Defense for Health Affairs
OCONUS	outside the continental United States
OIE	World Organization for Animal Health
OTSG	Office of the Army Surgeon General
PAHO	Pan American Health Organization
PCR	polymerase chain reaction
PI	pandemic influenza
PIPM	Pandemic Influenza Policy Model Extension
POM	Program Objective Memorandum
PPE	personal protective equipment
QA/QC	quality assurance/quality control
RSD	Research Sciences Department
RSV	respiratory syncytial virus
RTA	Royal Thai Army
RT-PCR	reverse transcription polymerase chain reaction
RVF	Rift Valley fever
SARS	severe acute respiratory syndrome
SEATO	Southeast Asia Treaty Organization
SME	subject matter expertise
SOP	standard operating procedure
SOUTHCOM	U.S. Southern Command
TMA	Tricare Management Activity
USACHPPM	U.S. Army Center for Health Promotion and Preventive Medicine
USAID	U.S. Agency for International Development
USAMC	U.S. Army Materiel Command
USAMRIID	United States Army Medical Research Institute for Infectious Diseases
USAMRMC	U.S. Army Medical Research and Materiel Command
USAMRU-K	U.S. Army Medical Research Unit, Kenya
USDA	U.S. Department of Agriculture
USDAAPHIS	U.S. Department of Agriculture's Animal and Plant Health Inspection Service
USG	United States government
USUHS	Uniformed Services University of the Health Sciences
UVRI	Uganda Virus Research Institute
VE	vaccine effectiveness
VRBPAC	Vaccines and Related Biological Products Advisory Committee
WARUN	Walter Reed/AFRIMS Research Unit Nepal
WHO	World Health Organization
WRAIR	Walter Reed Army Institute of Research
WRP	Walter Reed Project

Summary

The influenza pandemics of 1918, 1957, and 1968 offer a warning to the world about the potential dangers of the influenza virus. In 2006, after a series of cases and clusters of the highly pathogenic H5N1 avian virus made clear the threat of a possible pandemic, the U.S. Congress allocated $39 million to the Department of Defense Global Emerging Infections Surveillance and Response System (DoD-GEIS) to increase and improve its worldwide influenza surveillance network through upgrades to its domestic and overseas laboratories' capabilities.

Though the twentieth century saw the emergence of three influenza pandemics, the one that remains most widely researched is the 1918-1919 pandemic, commonly referred to as the "Spanish flu." This pandemic killed an estimated 50 million to 100 million people, thereby qualifying as the most deadly disease outbreak in history (Tumpey et al., 2005). In addition to the 1918 pandemic, the twentieth century experienced two other influenza pandemics which were milder and less devastating than the outbreak of 1918. The first of these occurred in 1957 and was known as the Asian flu pandemic (H2N2) (Potter, 2001). The Hong Kong pandemic of 1968, due to an antigenic shift to H3 (H3N2), was even milder than the 1957 pandemic, yet still reportedly killed half a million people worldwide (Dowdle, 1999; Kilbourne, 2006).

Almost three decades later, a new strain of influenza virus was discovered in China. Since 1997, the World Health Organization (WHO) has confirmed 318 human cases of H5N1 infection in 12 different countries, 192 of which were fatal (WHO, 2007). Approximately 150 million poultry have died since January 2004, either from the virus directly or as a result of culling efforts to contain the virus. H5N1 is already considered endemic in poultry in China, Vietnam, Thailand, Indonesia, and perhaps Cambodia and Laos (WHO, 2005).

The Executive Office of the President issued the Presidential Decision Directive NSTC-7 (National Science and Technology Council, Executive Office of the President, Presidential Decision Directive) in 1996, which declared that national and international capabilities for infectious disease surveillance, prevention, and response were inadequate to protect the health of U.S. citizens from emerging infectious diseases and called for a more robust national policy to improve these capabilities (IOM, 2001). This directive expanded the mission of the DoD to include support of global surveillance, training, research, and response to emerging infectious disease threats. In response to the NSTC-7 directive, DoD-GEIS was established in 1997 by the Assistant Secretary of Defense for Health Affairs to serve as the focal point for "initiating and coordinating the identification, reporting and responding to emerging infectious disease problems." GEIS is a tri-service program, and its activities are implemented within all three branches (Army, Navy, and Air Force) of the armed forces, although GEIS has no direct command authority over the facilities that implement its activities. The DoD overseas laboratories provide forward sites for GEIS activities. At present the DoD has five overseas laboratories: the U.S. Naval Medical Research Center Detachment (NMRCD) based in Lima, Peru; the U.S. Naval Medical Research Unit No. 2 (NAMRU-2) in Jakarta, Indonesia; the Armed Forces Research Institute of Medical Sciences (AFRIMS) in Bangkok, Thailand; the U.S. Naval Medical Research Unit No. 3 (NAMRU-3) in Cairo, Egypt; and the U.S. Army Medical Research Unit Kenya (USAMRU-K) in Nairobi. These laboratories, varying in size and capability, have field activities that operate in nearby countries and beyond, often with limited facilities within their regions of operation. In conjunction with the two domestic laboratories, the Naval Health Research Center in San Diego, California (NHRC) and the Air Force Institute for Operational Health in San Antonio, Texas (AFIOH), they work together to address the four stated goals of GEIS:

- Surveillance and detection
- Response and readiness
- Integration and innovation
- Cooperation and capacity building

Beginning with its creation in 1996, DoD-GEIS has focused on influenza, well aware of its potential to grow to pandemic proportions. The DoD-GEIS surveillance network was established to monitor host-country populations in areas where little was known about disease epidemiology, and this network currently includes patient enrollment sites in more than 20 countries in South America, the Middle East, sub-Saharan Africa, and central and southeast Asia (Canas et al., 2000). In a number of countries, including Indonesia, this DoD-GEIS network is the only way through which information on circulating influenza strains flows to WHO (Chretien et al., 2006a).

Between October 1, 2005 and February 28, 2006, the DoD-GEIS laboratories, working in conjunction with WHO, the Centers for Disease Control and Prevention (CDC), host country governments, and other key governmental and nongovernmental organizations, responded to 66 outbreaks in 22 countries worldwide. A number of these outbreak responses led to the identification of disease emergence or reemergence, notably influenza A (H5N1) in Egypt, Indonesia, Iraq, Kazakhstan, and Turkey. Additionally, the laboratories provide laboratory and field support, train host country and U.S. military medical personnel, and aid in the development of host country surveillance systems (Chretien et al., 2006b).

On January 2, 2005, the 109th Congress passed H.R. 1815, Sec. 748, "Pandemic Avian Flu Preparedness," which listed DoD-GEIS by name and called upon the secretary of defense to address ". . . surveillance efforts domestically and internationally." Subsequently, the DoD-GEIS was tasked by the assistant secretary of defense for health affairs to take the lead on the following activities laid out in Sec. 748, H.R. 1815:

- Surveillance efforts domestically and internationally, including those utilizing the Global Emerging Infections Systems (GEIS), and how such efforts are integrated with other ongoing surveillance systems
- Integration of pandemic and response planning with those of other federal departments, including the Department of Health and Human Services (HHS), Department of the Veterans Affairs, Department of State, and U.S. Agency for International Development
- Collaboration (as appropriate) with international entities engaged in pandemic preparedness and response

The congressional supplemental appropriation of $39.28 million associated with Sec. 748, H.R. 1815 was received by DoD-GEIS in March of 2006 and a variety of avian and pandemic influenza activities were implemented by DoD-GEIS-supported entities (Malone, 2005).

THE STUDY

An Institute of Medicine (IOM) committee was subsequently formed to evaluate the effectiveness of these laboratory-based programs in relation to the supplemental funding, and the report that follows details the committee's findings.

The committee that prepared this report, the Committee for the Assessment of DoD-GEIS Influenza Surveillance and Response Programs, was convened at the request of DoD-GEIS management to evaluate the execution of the fiscal year 2006 supplemental funding for avian influenza/pandemic influenza (AI/PI) surveillance and response. The committee was tasked with evaluating the DoD-GEIS AI/PI surveillance program for

a. the worth of each funded project's contribution to a comprehensive AI/PI surveillance program;
b. the adequacy of the program in view of the evolving epidemiologic factors;
c. responsiveness to the intent of Congress as expressed in Sec. 748, H.R.1815, Pandemic Avian Flu Preparedness;
d. consistency with the DoD and national plans; and
e. coordination of efforts with CDC, WHO, and local governments.

The committee focused its review on the development of conclusions and recommendations with long-term, program-level relevance as well as conclusions and recommendations regarding the improvement of specific DoD-GEIS projects. The committee used WHO and CDC guidelines as reference tools in conducting this review. Chapter 1, this report's introduction, offers a discussion of the committee's approach to addressing its charge along with additional background information regarding DoD-GEIS.

As part of this review, members of the committee visited NMRCD in Peru; NAMRU-2 in Indonesia; AFRIMS in Thailand; NAMRU-3 in Egypt; USAMRU-K in Kenya; the NHRC in San Diego, California; AFIOH in San Antonio, Texas; and DoD-GEIS Headquarters in Silver Spring, Maryland. Chapters 2 through 9 of this report present the committee's assessments of DoD-GEIS implementation at the overseas laboratories, at sites within the infrastructure of the military health system and at the DoD-GEIS headquarters. These chapters include discussions of each DoD unit's AI/PI activities as they related to management and planning, surveillance, response capacity, capacity building, and collaboration and coordination.[1] Chapter 10 of this report presents overarching conclusions and recommendations regarding DoD-GEIS's AI/PI activities as a whole. These overarching recommendations are excerpted and presented below as well. The boxes at the end of this summary provide, in brief, recommendations regarding the implementation of GEIS at the overseas laboratories, within the infrastruc-

[1]The chapters on the two domestic laboratories do not include sections on capacity building.

ture of the military health system and at the DoD-GEIS headquarters. By their very nature, recommendations focus on areas of program implementation where there is room for improvement. For a more complete picture of DoD-GEIS AI/PI activities, readers are encouraged to refer to chapters 1 through 10 of this report.

SUMMARY CONCLUSION

The Committee finds that DoD-GEIS has effectively executed and managed the fiscal year 2006 AI/PI supplemental funding, especially given the condensed timeframes that were available for planning and implementation. At DoD-GEIS headquarters as well as at the domestic and overseas laboratories, DoD-GEIS personnel absorbed the large increase in funding into programs aimed to successfully build DoD and host-country laboratory and human resource capacity, to globally expand information about avian influenza and acute respiratory diseases, to benefit the health of U.S. military personnel, and to strengthen U.S. relations within the global community.

SUMMARY OF RECOMMENDATIONS

Overarching Recommendations

Department of Defense Plans—Executive Agency

Before 1997 the DoD influenza surveillance program consisted largely of the surveillance program of the U.S. Air Force (AFIOH, 2006). With the establishment of GEIS in the late 1990s and, more recently, with the $39 million fiscal year 2006 avian influenza supplement, the program has grown to include efforts far beyond those of the historic Air Force program. These efforts include multimillion-dollar programs at the five DoD overseas labs and at the Naval Health Research Center in San Diego. Some of these new players have built enough independent laboratory capacity that they no longer are dependent on the laboratory services of the Air Force Institute for Operational Health (AFIOH). This has effectively moved AFIOH toward the margin. DoD-GEIS headquarters has the potential to provide unified technical and management oversight for DoD's integrated influenza and respiratory disease programs through a broad base of expertise and proximity to various service commands for the overseas labs, the Food and Drug Administration (FDA), and other federal agencies involved in influenza. The 2006 appropriations legislation[2] and DoD directives have already

[2] H.R. 1815, Sec. 748.

expanded the responsibility of DoD-GEIS headquarters for providing active project coordination and guidance across all DoD-GEIS-funded facilities. A multi-service executive agent has the potential to further improve the DoD influenza program, including maintaining consistency between DoD and national plans, limiting redundancy, and maximizing resources for AI/PI activities.

RECOMMENDATION 10-1. The executive agency functions of the DoD influenza and respiratory disease surveillance program should be reexamined in light of the evolution of the program in response to the potential of pandemic influenza. DoD-GEIS headquarters should be formally charged with providing managerial and technical oversight (quality assurance, safety, etc.) of the multi-service influenza and respiratory disease program and of the revised structure, including a codified chain of accountability.

Department of Defense Plans—DoD Communication and Coordination

The current level of collaboration among domestic and overseas laboratories and between the overseas laboratories and the DoD-GEIS headquarters is commendable, but it could be improved. Despite efforts to foster inter-laboratory dialogue and information sharing, certain laboratories appeared to be working in isolation and would benefit from additional information sharing and closer collaboration. Most laboratories are relatively new to the influenza field, and the learning curve over the past fiscal year has been steep.

RECOMMENDATION 10-2. Structured communication mechanisms should be established between DoD-GEIS headquarters and field sites (domestic and international) as well as among sites to create a functional network to enhance coordination of influenza and respiratory disease surveillance activities (epidemiologic, clinical, and laboratory) and to share best practices among all sites.

Each laboratory has learned valuable lessons in using the first year of the supplemental AI/PI funds, and, if shared, these lessons would greatly improve the continued program development of AI/PI activities at all DoD-GEIS sites. Increased inter-laboratory dialogue could decrease the likelihood of unintentional overlap of activities between different units and encourage more coordination of activities.

RECOMMENDATION 10-3. In Asia, the Naval Medical Research Unit No. 2 (Indonesia) and the Armed Forces Research Institute of

Medical Sciences (Thailand) should work together with DoD-GEIS headquarters to clarify the regional roles of each laboratory and to identify critical geographic areas requiring assistance to strengthen AI/PI surveillance programs in conjunction with World Health Organization and member states regional plans. The laboratories should coordinate the assignment of additional activities as well as prepare contingency plans to cover for each other in the event of a crisis (political, geologic, etc). The same recommendation applies to Africa and the roles of the Naval Medical Research Unit No. 3 (Egypt) and the U.S. Army Medical Research Unit-Kenya. DoD-GEIS headquarters should also work with the Naval Medical Research Center Detachment (Peru) to optimize its regional role in conjunction with Pan American Health Organization and member states regional plans.

National Plans

DoD-GEIS, through its AI/PI activities at the overseas laboratories and headquarters, has contributed greatly to the development of laboratory and communications infrastructures within partner countries. Beneficial effects can be seen from current DoD-GEIS efforts in 56 countries to assist its public health partners in building capacity through training and support of laboratory and communications infrastructures. In their continued implementation of AI/PI projects, GEIS headquarters and laboratories should consider the need to establish sustainable efforts to provide capacity to the host country even if funding is cut.

RECOMMENDATION 10-4. DoD-GEIS funding should be coordinated with funding from all sources to assure the likelihood that surveillance activities for influenza, other respiratory infections, and other emerging infections will be sustainable in overseas sites for the long term.

The Utility of Each Funded Project's Contribution to a Comprehensive AI/PI Surveillance Program

The DoD units were established at various times between 1942 and 1983, each with a fundamental mission of carrying out research relevant to the health of military personnel (DoD-GEIS, 2007). Over the years, the overseas laboratories have expanded their roles in host countries and in the surrounding geographic regions to include training activities and collaborative studies of pathogens of importance to the general public, but taking on a surveillance role, such as the AI/PI surveillance program, has been a significant departure from the historical research orientation. Strategic long-term planning for pandemic influenza-preparedness surveillance and response programs, supported by stable funding, would enable the DoD laboratories to determine the appropriate combination of research and public health surveillance needed to best meet the challenge of pandemic influenza as well as other possible emerging pathogens in their areas of responsibility.

RECOMMENDATION 10-5. DoD should issue a directive reaffirming that these traditionally research-oriented laboratories, particularly overseas, have a public health mission with respect to the host country and region; the directive should also provide strategic direction on the balance of military medicine-related research and public health activities.

Adequacy of the Program in View of Evolving Epidemiologic Factors—Human Influenza Surveillance

Using supplemental funding, DoD laboratories have established or improved influenza surveillance in all of their areas of responsibility. Acute respiratory diseases, including viral pathogens such as influenza, are of special interest to all militaries. The influenza pandemic of 1918 had a devastating impact upon military operations. One of the benefits of implementing a febrile respiratory infections surveillance and response program through a DoD entity is the strong relationship with the host-country military that DoD-GEIS laboratories can build upon. DoD-GEIS has opportunities to partner with militaries from host countries to improve surveillance capabilities and public health infrastructure (Chretien et al., 2007).

RECOMMENDATION 10-6. DoD-GEIS programs in the overseas laboratories should explore opportunities to develop or strengthen military influenza surveillance activities in collaboration with host-country military populations.

Adequacy of the Program in View of Evolving Epidemiologic Factors—Animal Influenza Surveillance

Most of the DoD-GEIS laboratories that received AI/PI supplemental funds are implementing animal surveillance programs, the majority of which are in wild bird populations. Despite the challenges, wild bird surveillance can, if done well, yield useful information on highly pathogenic influenza viruses. DoD-GEIS could provide valuable expertise at the country level in the integration of animal and human surveillance activities. Better coordination is needed at all levels between human surveillance activities and surveillance for influenza viruses in domestic birds (which have more opportunities to transmit influenza viruses to humans than do free flying birds) and in other animals.

RECOMMENDATION 10-7. DoD-GEIS headquarters should assess all of the current wild and domestic bird and animal surveillance activities and firmly establish goals, specifically targeting species and situations to fulfill these goals. DoD-GEIS headquarters and laboratories should seek collaborative opportunities to partner with organizations already studying influenza transmission in wild and domestic birds and animals in their areas.

Adequacy of the Program in View of Evolving Epidemiologic Factors—Laboratory

The AI/PI supplemental funding has been allocated to expanding or enhancing physical structure and laboratory capacity in all of the DoD-GEIS-supported sites. Many of the sites have used the supplemental funding to increase laboratory throughput, diagnostic capacity, and biosafety levels in order to manage highly pathogenic human and animal influenza A viruses, as well as to hire laboratory personnel.

RECOMMENDATION 10-8. To achieve successful influenza virus surveillance, each of the DoD overseas labs should have the capacity to provide reliable, definitive influenza diagnostic results in a safe and timely way.

Additionally, the expansion of laboratory capacity in domestic and overseas DoD laboratories has the potential to expand each laboratory's autonomy and self-sufficiency in terms of virus isolation and identification as well as in terms of decreasing the reliance on off-site and sometimes distant laboratory facilities.

RECOMMENDATION 10-9. In keeping with the goal of detecting newly recognized drifted or shifted influenza virus (or other emerging pathogens), the DoD-GEIS AI/PI surveillance system should be designed to capture influenza illness that could potentially present with different or unusual symptoms (e.g., conjunctivitis and diarrhea), bringing in outside help and support in the case of novel findings.

Adequacy of the Program in View of Evolving Epidemiologic Factors—Response Capacity

Laboratories must be prepared for expanded laboratory-based surveillance activities during this critical period between the initial epidemiologic harbingers of an influenza pandemic and eventual global spread. Laboratories currently testing a few samples a day, a week, or a month will be called upon to test many more during this period. Without necessarily adding new instruments or expanding in space, these laboratories could gear up to work more shifts if they could deploy trained lab technicians from other parts of the lab and rely upon sufficient supplies of reagents to perform the tests. Making the decision to redeploy technicians and work in shifts would be facilitated if labs have already devised a surge capacity plan, trained the other lab staff, and secured a source of reagents and supplies. Developing a surge capacity plan prior to human-to-human transmission could mean adapting to the increase in the number of samples in a few hours instead of days or weeks.

RECOMMENDATION 10-10. The DoD-GEIS influenza surveillance programs in the overseas laboratories should be complementary to the host-country laboratory system and help to increase surge capacity at the host country levels. DoD-GEIS should work with CDC, WHO, the U.S. Department of Agriculture, the Food and Agricultural Organization, and other entities at the headquarters and in-country levels to develop a plan to handle an increased number of influenza samples from humans or animals.

Adequacy of the Program in View of Evolving Epidemiologic Factors—Information Sharing

Current DoD-GEIS efforts to communicate influenza virus surveillance and other information within the DoD-GEIS consortium, within the DoD, to public health partners, and to the public are improving but remain insufficient. Of particular concern is the need for effective communication and dissemination of results as well as isolates at both the executive-agent and in-country levels. There must be a clear understanding of how and when information is to be communicated from the laboratories to WHO through the host country government and to the U.S. public health system via DoD. There is an established international system organized by WHO for flow of information and of influenza virus isolates from humans and animals. It was unclear in some places how DoD-GEIS laboratories were working with host governments to ensure that information was being fed into the WHO system. The channels of information flow from DoD-GEIS-supported activities and isolate distribution must be clearly understood by the host country and relevant international organizations.

RECOMMENDATION 10-11. DoD-GEIS influenza surveillance programs in the overseas laboratories in each host country should have a written understanding among all national and international partners delineating the reporting of influenza virus detections and the appropriate channels for exchanging isolates and communicating virological results. Such a document should include a clear statement of the laboratory designated by WHO as the reference laboratory for isolates from the host country.

Coordination and Collaboration—International Partners

While significant effort has been put into strengthening the coordination of avian and pandemic influenza activities, the overseas laboratories must continue their efforts to work within each country's national plan, thereby increasing national capacity and avoiding unintentionally working against the national plan. DoD influenza protocols should be executed in such a way that they cause a net strengthening of national and international capacity. As part of these collaborations, the overseas laboratories should also take opportunities to assist the host country in the development and implementation of disease-control guidelines and pandemic preparedness where appropriate and necessary. In some countries, for example, the committee found a lack of evidence at the local hospital level of influenza pandemic preparedness.

RECOMMENDATION 10-12. Overseas laboratories, with the strategic guidance of DoD-GEIS headquarters, should coordinate with national and regional influenza pandemic and enzootic response plans to establish the role for each laboratory in country and regionally. Where possible, DoD-GEIS laboratories should engage in host-country influenza coordinating activities, including tabletop response exercises and distribution of testing capacity, in concert with WHO and other international agencies. An important goal will be to strengthen linkages between laboratories and entities with key resources.

Coordination and Collaboration—U.S. Government Partners

DoD domestic and overseas laboratories have been working to improve their collaborations with other relevant U.S. agencies working in the same locations, including other DoD entities, CDC, the U.S. Agency for International Development (USAID), the U.S. Department of Agriculture

(USDA), and the National Aeronautics and Space Administration. The roles of various DoD laboratories in the event of a pandemic are less clear in the host country setting. The responsibilities of each U.S. government agency should be agreed upon by each U.S. agency and outlined by the host country government.

The relationship between the CDC and the DoD warrants particular attention. The CDC now has a presence in almost all of the countries where the overseas laboratories are located. In the past the DoD and the CDC have provided each other with backup support and entered into collaborative relationships on an as-needed basis. As influenza activities evolve, collaboration between the CDC and the DoD will be of utmost importance if both are to make efficient and effective use of limited resources. Similarly, strong relationships with other U.S. government partners such as USAID and USDA ensure most efficient use of U.S. funds.

RECOMMENDATION 10-13. DoD-GEIS should further strengthen its coordination and collaboration on pandemic influenza and other emerging infectious diseases with all U.S. partners, both domestically and in its overseas operations. These partners include HHS, CDC, the National Institutes of Health, FDA, USDA, the Department of State, the U.S. Agency for International Development, the Department of Homeland Security, and other relevant U.S. government efforts.

DEPARTMENT OF DEFENSE UNIT-SPECIFIC RECOMMENDATIONS

BOX S-1
Chapter 2 Recommendations
DoD-GEIS Headquarters

DoD-GEIS headquarters should strengthen its leadership role in the execution of DoD-GEIS influenza activities through strategic planning and distribution of future funding.

In order to assure the most effective use of the resources and varied expertise at the different DoD sites, mechanisms should be put into place to have systematic communication among the sites with respect to the various influenza-related projects and activities, including the development of a structured communication mechanism within each laboratory that would interact with headquarters to coordinate influenza activities, and the creation of regular opportunities for sharing of best practices facilitated by DoD-GEIS headquarters.

DoD-GEIS headquarters should continue to strengthen its in-house influenza expertise as necessary in order to give DoD laboratories and other relevant institutions the assistance needed to implement quality influenza surveillance and response activities.

DoD-GEIS headquarters should continue to work with U.S. and multilateral partners to ensure coordination among global influenza efforts.

BOX S-2
Chapter 3 Recommendations
Naval Medical Research Unit No. 2 Indonesia

NAMRU-2 should vigorously pursue work with novel findings that have a bearing on surveillance and the spread of virus, e.g., influenza/diarrheal studies.

NAMRU-2 should continue to strengthen its relationship with AFRIMS and to coordinate DoD-GEIS influenza activities in the region.

BOX S-3
Chapter 4 Recommendations
Armed Forces Research Institute of Medical Sciences Thailand

AFRIMS should establish more intensified surveillance for seasonal and novel strains of influenza at sites in temperate and tropical/subtropical parts of Nepal, in locales with commercial poultry production units, and at migratory bird resting sites.

AFRIMS should continue to work toward self-sufficiency in its isolation and identification systems in order to release PCR results more quickly to its national partners while taking appropriate steps to ensure laboratory containment and quality assurance.

AFRIMS should continue to provide relevant training, including epidemiological training, to U.S. and local personnel to enable its expansion of laboratory capabilities.

AFRIMS should continue to strengthen its relationship with NAMRU-2 in Indonesia and evaluate its roles in Asia and identify, where possible, critical geographic regions that are not covered by one or the other of these AI/PI programs.

BOX S-4
Chapter 5 Recommendations
Naval Medical Research Unit 3 Egypt

NAMRU-3 should prepare a short-term (2-3 years) strategic plan that identifies its priorities (surveillance/research and implementation/service delivery) in the AI/PI program and indicates NAMRU-3's role in the pre-pandemic stage.

NAMRU-3 should develop and implement a comprehensive information management system as soon as possible to prepare for the expanded needs that will be present during a potential pandemic and to improve routine information sharing in the EMRO region.

NAMRU-3 should assist the host country to develop the capacity to find emerging influenza pathogens beyond H5N1 and should integrate seasonal influenza and AI/PI programs as much as possible.

NAMRU-3 should explore opportunities to support the Ministry of Agriculture in increasing surveillance of domestic birds kept in homes and backyards.

NAMRU-3 should explore the expansion of laboratory capacity to include multiplex diagnostic equipment for respiratory diseases.

NAMRU-3 should develop a plan to expand its laboratory capacity in an early pandemic phase based on an assessment of how instrumentation and cross-training can be employed to optimize the laboratory and move from moderate throughput to high throughput with minimal staffing changes.

In order to assure the quality and sustainability of the regional influenza surveillance system, NAMRU-3 should work to establish standards and foundation documents for each of the steps in its laboratory-establishment process as well as to provide technical assistance for a new regional quality-assurance entity including (1) the development of a solid plan of strengthening regional countries' laboratory capacity with regard to avian influenza and maintaining this capacity through training, quality assurance, and proficiency testing; (2) continued collaboration with WHO to develop an external quality-assurance system for national central laboratories in the EMRO region; and (3) the use of NAMRU-3's extensive experience in capacity building (training, supervision, and mentoring) to develop structured (yet adaptable to each context) laboratory assessment checklists, training guidelines, and monitoring tools.

NAMRU-3 should continue to serve in a technical advisory role to the Egyptian Ministry of Health and carry out medical diplomacy by developing informal relationships with strategic partners while maintaining its role as an independent research agency with primary allegiances to the U.S. Navy.

NAMRU-3 should develop country- and region-specific 3-year strategies that focus on host sustainability as well as on the development, expansion, and maintenance of an influenza early warning system.

BOX S-5
Chapter 6 Recommendations
U.S. Army Medical Research Unit Kenya

The total number of adults and children each day who present to the clinics with acute respiratory illness for specimen collection under the current protocol should be logged, even though only five young children and five older children or adults will be sampled. By recording the total number of such patients and having the proportion of the five-patient samples that are positive, an estimate can be made of the burden of disease leading persons to seek attention at the sentinel health care facilities. Without collecting the number of syndromic eligible cases, burden cannot be estimated.

To foster collaboration and illustrate the value of the surveillance activities to stakeholders, USAMRU-K should consider supporting a weekly or biweekly summary of the number of cases of acute respiratory illness and of influenza virus isolations, by age group, to be sent to all the surveillance sites to provide feedback to the clinicians involved in the surveillance system.

USAMRU-K should draw on the experience of other DoD OCONUS laboratories in animal influenza surveillance. For example, the USAMRU-K veterinarian could be sent to NAMRU-2 in Indonesia to gain experience in performing tracheal cultures on trapped wild birds.

USAMRU-K should consider the expansion of laboratory capacity to include multitasking diagnostic equipment for respiratory diseases.

Based on the close proximity of laboratory space at KEMRI and the potential overlap in influenza activities, USAMRU-K should increase its efforts to facilitate communications between principal investigators at the USAMRU-K/NIC and CDC and the staff of the two laboratories, including joint seminars, data sharing, and cross training on equipment and BSL-3 principles and practices. As part of this communication, USAMRU-K and the NIC should develop a written understanding among all partners concerning WHO expectations about the reporting of influenza virus isolations and appropriate communication channels.

In order to maximize the AI/PI funds in Uganda, USAMRU-K should explore all options, including UVRI, in developing influenza virus diagnostic capacity within Uganda to ensure optimal use of national and external resources, promote collaboration among all sectors, and maximize potential for sustainability.

BOX S-6
Chapter 7 Recommendations
Naval Medical Research Center Detachment Peru

NMRCD should continue to work to increase information sharing with both the DoD-GEIS headquarters staff and staff at other overseas laboratories.

NMRCD should support additional tabletop simulation exercises in which NMRCD has the potential to identify areas of the Peruvian plan that need strengthening.

NMRCD should consider expanding its surveillance activities to include populations at high risk of contracting avian influenza, including poultry farm workers, live bird market workers, and military training camps.

In conjunction with improved sharing of facilities for testing avian viruses at SENASA, NMRCD should develop mechanisms to enable testing of avian and human influenza isolates in separate laboratory facilities and plan to obtain resources to expand its BSL-3 laboratory, including showering-out facilities.

NMRCD should continue to support in-house and webcast training in epidemiological surveillance and laboratory methods. Outbreak response should receive additional emphasis, including Peru's Field Epidemiology Training Program.

A close working relationship, the sharing of facilities, the training of technicians, the sharing of specimens, support for maintenance, support to meet cold-chain needs, and other forms of integration with the INS and SENASA laboratories should continue to be cultivated by NMRCD. A common surveillance database with both NMRCD and INS results would be desirable.

BOX S-7
Chapter 8 Recommendations
Naval Health Research Center San Diego

NHRC should investigate factors contributing to the ability or inability of the eight military training sites to meet maximum FRI surveillance targets as well as continue to explore methods to validate the reliability of virus-effectiveness data, which are available from no other populations on a consistent basis.

The services should explore interpretation of the syndromic surveillance mandate to include laboratory diagnostic testing of clinically ill subjects in order to facilitate crucial febrile respiratory illness and other infectious disease surveillance in military populations.

The NHRC team should look into other virus culture methods to speed isolation.

BOX S-8
Chapter 9 Recommendations
Air Force Institute for Operational Health San Antonio

AFIOH's influenza program should employ a strong doctoral-level molecular biologist with demonstrated technical and leadership skills. These should include a strong background in laboratory quality control methods. The program staff should be well-versed in the data analytic approaches desired by the FDA influenza vaccine committee. The laboratory should regularly obtain technical guidance from appropriate sources (e.g., CDC, FDA, academia, and GEIS headquarters) to ensure that it is using state-of-the-art methods and is targeting appropriate specimen sources.

In order to minimize potential for contamination in the molecular biology section and to improve the data generated by this section, AFIOH should seek expertise in molecular biology techniques and their implementation in a diagnostic laboratory setting.

AFIOH should consider the expansion of its laboratory capacity to include multitasking diagnostic equipment for respiratory diseases.

AFIOH should create a sustainable and useful archive of the original patient sample and virus isolate materials in this laboratory to ensure this national resource can be used to fulfill the missions of the DoD-GEIS AI/PI program.

AFIOH should collaborate with both the National Institutes of Health and Los Alamos National Laboratory, and provide sequencing data and samples when appropriate.

AFIOH should seek out cutting-edge academic collaborators in order to expand the methodologies available to identify agents responsible for mixed infections, which could possibly result in the identification of new agents responsible for respiratory infections.

AFIOH should continue to conduct periodic training exercises and dry runs in order to further develop and test the surge plan.

In conjunction with DoD-GEIS headquarters, AFIOH should examine the current activities at AFIOH, and strategies for strengthening the AFIOH operations should be identified and supported.

REFERENCES

Air Force Institute for Operational Health. 2006. *The Department of Defense Global Laboratory-Based Influenza Surveillance Program: FY 2006 annual report.* San Antonio.

Canas, L. C., K. Lohman, J. A. Pavlin, T. Endy, D. L. Singh, P. Pandey, M. P. Shrestha, R. M. Scott, K. L. Russell, D. Watts, M. Hajdamowicz, I. Soriano, R. W. Douce, J. Neville, and J. C. Gaydos. 2000. The Department of Defense laboratory-based global influenza surveillance system. *Military Medicine* 165(7 Suppl. 2):52-56.

Chretien, J. P., J. C. Gaydos, J. L. Malone, and D. L. Blazes. 2006a. Global network could avert pandemics. *Nature* 440(7080):25-26.

Chretien, J. P., D. L. Blazes, J. C. Gaydos, S. A. Bedno, R. L. Coldren, R. C. Culpepper, D. J. Fyrauff, K. C. Earhart, M. M. Mansour, J. S. Glass, M. D. Lewis, B. L. Smoak, and J. L. Malone, 2006b. Experience of a global laboratory network in responding to infectious disease epidemics. *Lancet Infectious Diseases* 6(9):538-540.

Chretien, J. P., D. L. Blazes, R. L. Coldren, M. D. Lewis, J. Gaywee, K. Kana, N. Sirisopana, V. Vallejos, C. C. Mundaca, S. Montano, G. J. Martin, and J. C. Gaydos. 2007. The importance of militaries from developing countries in global infectious disease surveillance. *Bulletin of the World Health Organization* 85(3):174-180.

DoD-GEIS (Department of Defense Global Emerging Infections System). 2007. *DoD-GEIS website.* http://www.geis.fhp.osd.mil/ (accessed August 7, 2007).

Dowdle, W. R. 1999. Influenza A virus recycling revisited. *Bulletin of the World Health Organization* 77(10):820-828.

IOM (Institute of Medicine). 2001. *Perspectives on the Department of Defense Global Emerging Infections Surveillance and Response System: A program review.* Washington, DC: National Academy Press.

Kilbourne, E. D. 2006. Influenza pandemics of the 20th century. *Emerging Infectious Diseases* 12(1):9-14.

Malone, J. L. 2005. Fiscal Year 2006 Special supplemental budget for Pandemic Influenza Preparedness Memorandum. *Memorandum for DoD-GEIS-supported laboratories and DoD agencies.* December 22, 2005.

Potter, C. W. 2001. A history of influenza. *Journal of Applied Microbiology* 91(4):572-579.

Tumpey, T. M., C. F. Basler, P. V. Aguilar, H. Zeng, A. Solorzano, D. E. Swayne, N. J. Cox, J. M. Katz, J. K. Taubenberger, P. Palese, and A. Garcia-Sastre. 2005. Characterization of the reconstructed 1918 Spanish influenza pandemic virus. *Science* 310(5745):77-80.

WHO. 2005. *Avian influenza frequently asked questions.* http://www.who.int/csr/disease/avian_influenza/avian_faqs/en/index.html (accessed July 27, 2007).

WHO. 2007. *Cumulative number of confirmed human cases of avian influenza A/(H5N1) reported to WHO.* http://www.who.int/csr/disease/avian_influenza/country/cases_table_2007_07_25/en/index.html (accessed July 27, 2007).

1

Introduction

BACKGROUND

The influenza pandemic of 1918 offers a warning to the world about the potential dangers of the influenza virus. Of all the influenza pandemics that have appeared in recorded history, the 1918 pandemic was particularly devastating. It killed an estimated 650,000 Americans (Tumpey et al., 2005), and for several weeks in October 1918 it was causing 5,000 to 6,000 deaths each week in the U.S. Army (Crosby, 1989).

In 2006, after a series of H5N1 avian influenza virus infections and deaths among people in Asia and Africa raised the threat of a possible pandemic, the U.S. Congress allocated $39 million to the Department of Defense Global Emerging Infections Surveillance and Response System (DoD-GEIS) to increase and improve its worldwide influenza surveillance network through upgrades of DoD domestic and overseas public health surveillance and laboratory capabilities. An Institute of Medicine (IOM) committee was subsequently formed to evaluate the effectiveness of these laboratory-based surveillance programs in relation to the supplemental funding. This report describes the committee's findings.

Three major influenza pandemics emerged in the twentieth century, one of which—the pandemic of 1918-1919, commonly referred to as the "Spanish flu"—killed an estimated 50 million to 100 million people, thereby making it the most deadly known disease outbreak in history. The first wave of the pandemic in the United States arrived in the spring of 1918, followed by two subsequent, more deadly waves in the fall of 1918 and the winter of 1918-1919 (Taubenberger and Morens, 2006). Retrospectively, the earliest cases seen in the United States appeared in the U.S. military.

The strain of influenza responsible for the 1918 pandemic was particularly deadly, with a fatality rate of roughly 2 percent as compared with a fatality rate of around 0.1 percent for contemporary strains of influenza virus (IOM, 2004). The 1918 pandemic also exhibited an unprecedented excess of mortality among people from 20 to 40 years old, a population that has historically demonstrated a low influenza mortality rate, both in the years prior to 1918 and the years since (Morens and Fauci, 2007). Military populations in particular were severely affected by the 1918 pandemic.

The genome of the 1918 influenza virus has been recently sequenced from RNA fragments obtained from archival and frozen lung tissue of viral pneumonia victims. From that analysis the extinct pandemic strain of 1918 was identified as an influenza A virus, subtype H1N1. Studies under high-containment conditions using the reconstructed 1918 virus showed a high fatality rate in animal models 3 to 4 days after infection, a characteristic not described for any other human influenza virus (Tumpey et al., 2005).

The two other major influenza pandemics of the twentieth century were milder and less devastating than the 1918 pandemic. The first of these was the Asian flu pandemic of 1957-1958 caused by subtype H2N2. The virus, first found in the Far East, was identified in the United States in June 1957, with the first outbreak occurring in September and the peak coming in October. The timing of the epidemics coincided with the opening of the winter school term (Payne, 1958). A second wave hit in early 1958. Fatalities occurred mainly among the very young and the very old and in total claimed the lives of roughly 1,000,000 people (Potter, 2001).

The pandemic of 1968, caused by an H3N2 strain descended from H2N2 by antigenic shift (genetic reassortment), was milder than the 1957 pandemic, yet it still was estimated to have caused 500,000 deaths worldwide. The new strain was first isolated in Hong Kong in July 1968, although it most likely originated in nearby Guangdong Province, China. The pandemic proved less deadly in the United States than expected. Experts have suggested a variety of possible reasons: (1) antigenic overlap with the neuraminidase of the earlier H2N2 dominant strain, which would have provided a degree of cross protection; (2) the presence of preexisting antibodies (and protection) among the elderly born prior to 1893 as a result of the 1889-1891 pandemic; (3) the fact that the pandemic peaked around the holiday season in December, a time when most children are temporarily out of school, which would have slowed the spread of the virus; and (4) improvements in medical care and access to effective treatment (Dowdle, 1999; Kilbourne, 2006).

In 1977, an H1N1 virus reemerged in the Far East, genetically closely related to strains prevalent in the late (~1950) H1N1 era (Nakajima et al.,

1978). Though the origin of the virus remains in question, it met the basic criteria of a pandemic strain in that a significant percentage of the population (those people born after 1956) had no immunity and there was rapid global transmission. However, it differed from previous pandemics in that the disease was mild and most persons older than 20 years of age were protected through previous immunologic experience with the H1N1 subtype. The H1N1 subtype continues to co-circulate with H3N2. The genetic identity of the 1977 virus with strains from the late H1N1 era (~1950) strongly suggested that this virus had reappeared (Kendal et al., 1978; Nakajima et al., 1978). The reason for this is unexplained.

In 1996 a highly pathogenic H5N1 avian influenza virus was isolated from farmed geese in Guangdong Province, China. In the following year reports from Hong Kong described outbreaks first in farm chickens and then in live poultry markets. Eighteen cases of human infection were reported, six of which were fatal, providing the first documented instance of a purely avian influenza virus causing respiratory disease and death in humans (Claas et al., 1998; WHO, 2007a). While the H5N1 virus of 1997 has not been detected subsequent to the culling of poultry in Hong Kong, the precursor virus found in the Guangdong geese in 1996 persisted in southern China; it has subsequently gone on to exchange various genes over time with unspecified avian influenza viruses to produce a series of highly pathogenic H5N1 descendants, some of which have spread to other parts of Asia, Europe, and northern Africa (Ducatez et al., 2006; Salzberg et al., 2007; Smith et al., 2006) (see Figure 1-1).

From 2003 to writing of this report in July 2007, the WHO had confirmed a total of 319 human cases of H5N1 infection in 12 different countries, 192 of which were fatal (fatality rate around 60 percent) (WHO, 2007b). Approximately 150 million poultry have died since January 2004, either from the virus itself or as a result of culling aimed at containing the virus. H5N1 is considered endemic in poultry in China, Vietnam, Thailand, Indonesia, Egypt, Nigeria, and perhaps Cambodia and Laos (WHO, 2005; FAO, 2007).

Historically, the U.S. military has played an important international role in influenza virus surveillance and vaccine development (Woodward, 1994). In 1941, on the eve of the U.S. entry into World War II, concern about a repeat of the 1918 influenza pandemic and its disastrous effects on armed forces led the U.S. military to establish a commission on influenza and place highest priority on rapid development of an effective influenza vaccine. The first successful large-scale influenza vaccine field trials anywhere in the world were completed by the commission in 1943 (Francis, 1954). In 1954 the Department of Defense issued an influenza immunization policy that mandated quick pandemic risk assessment along with the formulation and provision of vaccines in order to protect military person-

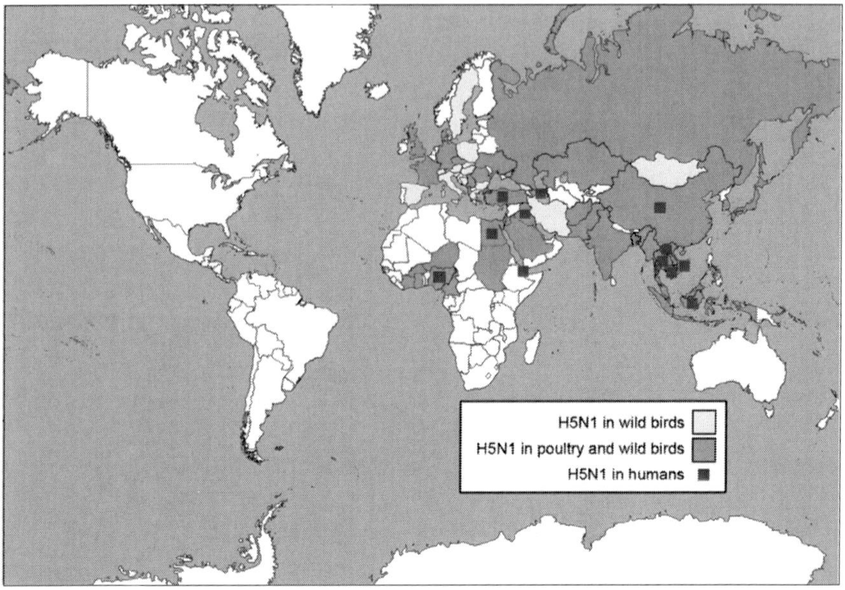

FIGURE 1-1 Nations with confirmed cases H5N1 avian influenza.
SOURCE: U.S. Fish and Wildlife Service, 2007.

nel. In 1957 and again in 1968, the U.S. Military Commission on Influenza provided crucial international leadership in surveillance and risk assessment in response to reports of potential influenza pandemics emerging in the Far East. Candidate strains isolated by the military or obtained through its overseas contacts greatly accelerated production and provision of vaccines in both pandemics.

In 1996, the Executive Office of the President issued the presidential decision directive NSTC-7 (NSTC is the National Science and Technology Council of the Executive Office of the President), which declared that both the international and domestic capabilities for emerging infectious disease surveillance, prevention, and response were inadequate to protect U.S. citizens from such threats (NSTC, 1996). To address that issue, NSTC-7 expanded the mission of the DoD to include support of global surveillance, training, research, and response to emerging infectious disease threats. The DoD was to "strengthen its global disease reduction efforts through centralized coordination; improved preventive health programs and epidemiologic capabilities; and enhanced involvement with military treatment facilities and overseas laboratories" (NSTC, 1996). NSTC-7 also called for increased communication and coordination among U.S. government agencies with responsibilities for addressing emerging infectious diseases.

GEIS, established by the Assistant Secretary of Defense for Health Affairs in 1996 in response to NSTC-7, was tasked with "initiating and coordinating the identification, reporting and responding to emerging infectious disease problems" (Bancroft and Schlagel, 1997). GEIS is a tri-service program, and its activities are implemented within all three branches of the Armed Forces (Army, Navy, and Air Force), although GEIS has no direct command authority over the facilities where its activities are implemented (DoD-GEIS, 2006).

The history of U.S. overseas military medical research goes back more than a century to the days of Walter Reed work on yellow fever epidemiology in Cuba at the turn of the 20th century (IOM, 2001). The current network of DoD overseas medical research units began with the establishment of the U.S. Navy Medical Research Unit in Egypt in 1942. (Gambel and Hibbs, 1996). These DoD overseas laboratories provide forward sites for GEIS activities. The DoD currently has five overseas medical research units and three domestic medical research/public health laboratories with a major focus on influenza (see Table 1-1): the U.S. Naval Medical Research No. 2 (NAMRU-2) in Jakarta, In-

TABLE 1-1 Primary DoD Overseas and Domestic Laboratories Receiving DoD-GEIS AI/PI Funding

Laboratory	Location	Date Established
Naval Medical Research Unit No. 2 (NAMRU-2)	Jakarta, Indonesia	1970
Armed Forces Research Institute of Medical Sciences (AFRIMS)	Bangkok, Thailand	1958
Naval Medical Research Unit No. 3 (NAMRU-3)	Cairo, Egypt	1942
U.S. Army Medical Research Unit (USAMRU-K)	Nairobi, Kenya	1969
Naval Medical Research Center Detachment (NMRCD)	Lima, Peru	1983
Naval Health Research Center (NHRC)	San Diego, Calif.	1996[a]
Air Force Institute for Operational Health (AFIOH)	San Antonio, Tex.	1976

[a]Naval Respiratory Disease Laboratory (NRDL) was established in 1996 as one of six departments of the Naval Health Research Center (NHRC).

SOURCE: Adapted from: DoD-GEIS Website http://www.geis.fhp.osd.mil/. NHRC information adapted from FY06 Annual Summary Report, NHRC.

donesia; the Armed Forces Research Institute of Medical Sciences (AFRIMS) in Bangkok, Thailand; the U.S. Naval Medical Research Unit No. 3 (NAMRU-3) in Cairo, Egypt; the U.S. Army Medical Research Unit-Kenya (USAMRU-K) in Nairobi; the U.S. Naval Medical Research Center Detachment (NMRCD) based in Lima, Peru; the Naval Health Research Center in San Diego (NHRC); the Air Force Institute for Operational Health in San Antonio (AFIOH); and the U.S. Army Medical Research Institute of Infectious Diseases in Fort Detrick (USAMRIID).

The work of these five overseas laboratories is considerable and includes basic and applied research; public health surveillance; capacity building in the host countries by training scientists and developing laboratories and institutions; and, upon request, the provision of assistance to host countries during humanitarian emergencies (Gambel and Hibbs, 1996). These laboratories, varying in size and capability, have field activities that operate in other nearby countries and beyond, often with limited facilities within their regions of operation. Together with the three domestic DoD-GEIS-affiliated medical laboratories they work to address the four stated goals of GEIS:

- Surveillance and detection
- Response and readiness
- Integration and innovation
- Cooperation and capacity building

In relation to these four goals, GEIS monitors all infectious diseases in military forces, with respiratory diseases, especially influenza, gastrointestinal infections, and febrile illness syndromes, primarily dengue and malaria, included among the priority surveillance operations. Since its formation in 1997, GEIS has maintained a focus on surveillance and respiratory diseases. The $39 million Congressional Supplement allocated in fiscal year 2006 by HR 2863 for pandemic and avian influenza—which in turn prompted the IOM evaluation detailed in this report—represented a fivefold increase in the annual GEIS budget and significantly enhanced the operations of both the GEIS-affiliated overseas and domestic laboratories (DoD-GEIS, 2006).

More specifically, HR 2863 allowed DoD-GEIS to address the following goals:

- Increase worldwide surveillance
- Upgrade existing surveillance
- Upgrade laboratory capability
- Establish a surveillance information network among all elements (Erickson, 2006)

The worth of these overseas laboratories has been considered by a variety of related parties, and they have consistently concluded that the laboratories and the network that they form play an important role in addressing the challenges that emerging infectious diseases present to the international community, particularly those in developing countries that lack basic laboratories and epidemiologic capabilities. In a 2006 article published in *Lancet Infectious Diseases*, a global network of broad-based laboratories was proposed as a way to address some of these challenges, and the five DoD military overseas laboratories were offered as the model for this new network, perhaps due in part to the unique advantages and capabilities they offer. "Access to the natural environments in which diseases occur is crucial if research to prevent and control infectious diseases is to progress, and if tools, such as diagnostics, vaccines, and chemoprophylactic agents . . . are to be properly tested" (Gambel and Hibbs, 1996).

Beginning with its creation in 1996, DoD-GEIS has focused on influenza, well aware of its potential to grow to pandemic proportions. The DoD-GEIS influenza surveillance network was established to monitor host-country populations in areas where little was known about disease epidemiology, and this network currently includes patient-enrollment sites in more than 20 countries in South America, the Middle East, sub-Saharan Africa, and central and southeast Asia (Canas et al., 2000). In a number of countries, including Indonesia, this DoD-GEIS network is a key way through which information on circulating influenza strains flows to the World Health Organization (WHO) (Chretien et al., 2006a). The importance of military laboratories was also noted in a 1998 WHO report, which summarized the findings of three surveys conducted to evaluate the possibility of including military laboratories in the WHO network and concluded that "a wealth of information is obtained by military laboratories and health-care facilities on populations at high risk for infectious diseases" (D'Amelio and Heymann, 1998).

Between October 1, 2003, and February 28, 2006, the DoD-GEIS laboratories, working in conjunction with the WHO, the Centers for Disease Control and Prevention (CDC), host country governments, and other key governmental and nongovernmental organizations, responded to 66 outbreaks in 22 countries worldwide. A number of these outbreak responses led to the identification of disease emergence or reemergence, notably influenza A (H5N1) in Egypt, Indonesia, Iraq, Kazakhstan, and Turkey. Additionally, they provide laboratory and field support, train host-country and U.S. military medical personnel, and aid in the development of host-country surveillance systems (Chretien et al., 2006b).

Military forces in a number of developing countries work closely with their ministries of health to help to strengthen their infectious disease surveillance and control programs. In turn, a number of activities performed by the DoD overseas laboratories are done so in collaboration with the host-country military, and two of these five laboratories are hosted by the foreign militaries: the Peruvian Navy hosts NMRCD in Lima and the Royal Thai Army (RTA) hosts AFRIMS in Bangkok. Examples of their collaborative efforts include a unit-based surveillance system developed by RTA and AFRIMS to improve infectious disease surveillance in remote areas of Thailand along the country's borders with Cambodia and the Lao People's Democratic Republic and also an electronic disease surveillance system, Alerta, developed by the Peruvian Navy and NMRCD. Before the development of this system, the Peruvian Navy had relied on a time-consuming paper-based reporting system (Chretien et al., 2007).

CHARGE TO THE COMMITTEE

The Department of Defense requested that an IOM committee conduct an evaluation of what has been done in the Avian Influenza Surveillance and Response effort in fiscal year 2006 and fiscal year 2007 under the DoD-GEIS program. The committee was directed to provide advice on improving surveillance and response efforts in fiscal years 2006-2008 and to recommend additional surveillance and response efforts that could be undertaken to enhance the likelihood of early detection and timely response to an influenza pandemic. The committee was also required to provide recommendations for changes in support of surveillance and research related to avian influenza and pandemic influenza (AI/PI) preparedness and response. And, in addition, the committee was to perform site visits to DoD elements in receipt of DoD-GEIS AI/PI surveillance funding, including the five overseas DoD medical research laboratories (Bangkok, Jakarta, Cairo, Nairobi, and Lima), the Air Force Institute for Operational Health (AFIOH) in San Antonio, and the Naval Health Research Center (NHRC) in San Diego.

Specifically, the evaluation of the DoD-GEIS AI/PI surveillance program was to address the following:

(a) The utility of each funded project's contribution to a comprehensive AI/PI surveillance program

(b) The adequacy of the program in view of the evolving epidemiologic factors

(c) Responsiveness to the intent of Congress as expressed in Sec. 748, HR1815, Pandemic Avian Flu Preparedness

(d) Consistency with the DoD and national plans

(e) Coordination of efforts with the Centers for Disease Control and Prevention, the World Health Organization, and local governments

THE STUDY PROCESS

At the request of GEIS management, the IOM convened a committee, the Committee for the Assessment of DoD-GEIS Influenza Surveillance and Response Programs. The study began in December 2006, with a meeting held in Washington, D.C., to familiarize the committee with GEIS, its use of the supplemental funding, its related priorities and goals, its coordination with other organizations, governments, national plans, and so forth. This committee meeting, which was open to the public, involved representatives from GEIS headquarters, NHRC and AFIOH, and a number of other institutions, including CDC, the Office of the Assistant Secretary of Defense for Health Affairs, the Homeland Security Council of the White House, the Department of Infectious Diseases at St. Jude Children's Research Hospital, and the Food and Drug Administration.

Thereafter, committee members made site visits to recipients of the GEIS AI/PI supplement, including the five DoD overseas laboratories and NHRC and AFIOH. In March 2007, teams of two or three committee members each visited NMRCD in Lima; NAMRU-2 in Jakarta plus a trip to Phnom Penh, Cambodia; AFRIMS in Bangkok plus a trip to Kathmandu, Nepal; NAMRU-3 in Cairo; the USAMRU-K field site in Kisumu, Kenya plus a trip to Entebbe, Uganda; NHRC in San Diego; and AFIOH in San Antonio. Lastly, a delegation of committee members participated in a meeting at GEIS Headquarters in Silver Spring, MD, where they were able to discuss in detail the management and oversight roles of that office.

The visits lasted approximately five days at each overseas laboratory and two days at each domestic lab. Each member of the committee participated in at least one visit. During these visits, committee members toured laboratory facilities, attended briefings and presentations, and met with laboratory staff and collaborators, including representatives from CDC, WHO, national ministries of health, and local hospitals and public health laboratories. In total, eight site visits and three committee meetings (one of which was open to the public) were held during the course of the study.

The committee focused its review on the development of conclusions and recommendations with long-term, program-level relevance as well as the improvement of specific DoD-GEIS projects. The committee used WHO and CDC guidelines as reference tools in conducting this review.[1]

In the remainder of this report, chapters 2 through 9 present the

---

[1]Overview of WHO Framework for Monitoring & Evaluating Surveillance and Response Systems for Communicable Diseases; Updated Guidelines for Evaluating Public Health Surveillance Systems; Influenza Pandemic Plan: The Role of WHO and Guidelines for National and Regional Planning.

committee's assessments of DoD-GEIS implementation at the DoD-GEIS headquarters, at overseas laboratories, and at sites within the military health system. These chapters include discussions of the individual DoD units' pandemic/avian influenza activities as they relate to management and planning, surveillance, response capacity, capacity building, and collaboration and coordination.[2] A final chapter provides summary conclusions and recommendations regarding DoD-GEIS's AI/PI activities as a whole.

REFERENCES

Bancroft, W. H., and C. Schlagel. 1997. *Implementation of DoD emerging infectious disease surveillance and response system.* Memorandum for Commander, U.S. Army Medical Research and Materiel Command, Commanding Officer, U.S. Naval Medical Research and Development Command. Department of the Army, U.S. Department of Defense, Ft. Detrick, Md., June 9, 1997. On file with the National Academies Public Access Records Office.

Canas, L. C., K. Lohman, J. A. Pavlin, T. Endy, D. L. Singh, P. Pandey, M. P. Shrestha, R. M. Scott, K. L. Russell, D. Watts, M. Hajdamowicz, I. Soriano, R. W. Douce, J. Neville, and J. C. Gaydos. 2000. The Department of Defense laboratory-based global influenza surveillance system. *Military Medicine* 165(7 Suppl. 2):52-56.

Chretien, J. P., J. C. Gaydos, J. L. Malone, and D. L. Blazes. 2006a. Global network could avert pandemics. *Nature* 440(7080):25-26.

Chretien, J. P., D. L. Blazes, J. C. Gaydos, S. A. Bedno, R. L. Coldren, R. C. Culpepper, D. J. Fyrauff, K. C. Earhart, M. M. Mansour, J. S. Glass, M. D. Lewis, B. L. Smoak, and J. L. Malone, 2006b. Experience of a global laboratory network in responding to infectious disease epidemics. *Lancet Infectious Diseases* 6(9):538-540.

Chretien, J. P., D. L. Blazes, R. L. Coldren, M. D. Lewis, J. Gaywee, K. Kana, N. Sirisopana, V. Vallejos, C. C. Mundaca, S. Montano, G. J. Martin, and J. C. Gaydos. 2007. The importance of militaries from developing countries in global infectious disease surveillance. *Bulletin of the World Health Organization* 85(3):174-180.

Claas, E. C., A. D. Osterhaus, R. van Beek, J. C. De Jong, G. F. Rimmelzwaan, D. A. Senne, S. Krauss, K. F. Shortridge, and R. G. Webster. 1998. Human influenza A H5N1 virus related to a highly pathogenic avian influenza virus. *Lancet* 351(9101):472-477.

Crosby, A. 1989. *America's forgotten pandemic.* Cambridge, England: Cambridge University Press.

D'Amelio, R., and D. L. Heymann. 1998. Can the military contribute to global surveillance and control of infectious diseases? *Emerging Infectious Diseases* 4(4):704-705.

DoD-GEIS (Department of Defense Global Emerging Infections System). 2006. *DoD Global Emerging Infections Surveillance and Response System annual report fiscal year 2006.* Silver Spring, MD: Walter Reed Army Institute for Research

Dowdle, W. R. 1999. Influenza A virus recycling revisited. *Bulletin of the World Health Organization* 77(10):820-828.

Ducatez, M. F., C. M. Olinger, A. A. Owoade, S. De Landtsheer, W. Ammerlaan, H. G. Niesters, A. D. Osterhaus, R. A. Fouchier, and C. P. Muller. 2006. Multiple introductions of H5N1 in Nigeria. *Nature* 442(7098):37.

[2]The chapters on the two domestic laboratories do not include sections on capacity building.

Erickson, R. L. 2006. *The DoD-GEIS influenza surveillance and response programs: Charge to the IOM committee.* PowerPoint presentation at first meeting of the IOM Committee for the Assessment of DoD-GEIS, December 19, Washington, D.C.

FAO (Food and Agricultural Organization of the United Nations). 2007. *Combining poultry vaccination with other disease control measures to combat H5N1.* http://www.fao.org/newsroom/en/news/2007/1000527/index.html (accessed July 27, 2007).

Francis, T. 1954. Vaccination against influenza. In *Influenza, a review of current research.* Ed. by WHO. Geneva: World Health Organization. Pp. 125-140.

Gambel, J. M. and R. G. Hibbs, Jr. 1996. U.S. military overseas medical research laboratories. *Military Medicine* 161(11):638-645.

IOM (Institute of Medicine). 2001. *Perspectives on the Department of Defense Global Emerging Infections Surveillance and Response System: A program review.* Washington, DC: National Academy Press.

IOM. 2004. *The threat of pandemic influenza: Are we ready?* Washington, DC: The National Academies Press.

Kendal, A. P., G. R. Noble, J. J. Skehel, and W. R. Dowdle. 1978. Antigenic similarity of influenza A (H1N1) viruses from epidemics in 1977-1978 to Scandinavian strains isolated in epidemics of 1950-1951. *Virology* 89(2):632-636.

Kilbourne, E. D. 2006. Influenza pandemics of the 20th century. *Emerging Infectious Diseases* 12(1):9-14.

Morens, D. M., and A. S. Fauci. 2007. The 1918 influenza pandemic: Insights for the 21st century. *Journal of Infectious Diseases* 195(7):1018-1028.

Nakajima, K., U. Desselberger, and P. Palese. 1978. Recent human influenza A (H1N1) viruses are closely related genetically to strains isolated in 1950. *Nature* 274(5669):334-339.

NSTC (National Science and Technology Council, Executive Office of the President). 1996. *Presidential decision directive NSTC-7: Emerging infections.* Washington, DC: National Science and Technology Council, Executive Office of the President.

Payne, A. M. 1958. Some aspects of the epidemiology of the 1957 influenza pandemic. *Journal of the Royal Society of Medicine.* 51(12):1009-1015.

Potter, C. W. 2001. A history of influenza. *Journal of Applied Microbiology* 91(4):572-579.

Salzberg, S. L., C. Kingsford, G. Cattoli, D. J. Spiro, D. A. Janies, M. M. Aly, I. H. Brown, E. Couacy-Hymann, G. M. De Mia, H. D. Do, A. Guercio, T. Joannis, A. S. M. Ali, A. Osmani, I. Padalino, M. D. Saad, V. Savic, N. A. Sengamalay, S. Yingst, J. Zaborsky, O. Zorman-Rojs, E. Ghedin, and I. Capua. 2007. Genome analysis linking recent European and African influenza (H5N1) viruses. *Emerging Infectious Diseases* 13(5):713-718.

Smith, G. J., X. H. Fan, J. Wang, K. S. Li, K. Qin, J. X. Zhang, D. Vijaykrishna, C. L. Cheung, K. Huang, J. M. Rayner, J. S. Peiris, H. Chen, R. G. Webster, and Y. Guan. 2006. Emergence and predominance of an H5N1 influenza variant in China. *Proceedings of the National Academy of Science of the USA* 103(45):16936-16941.

Taubenberger, J. K., and D. M. Morens. 2006. 1918 influenza: The mother of all pandemics. *Emerging Infectious Diseases* 12(1):15-22.

Tumpey, T. M., C. F. Basler, P. V. Aguilar, H. Zeng, A. Solorzano, D. E. Swayne, N. J. Cox, J. M. Katz, J. K. Taubenberger, P. Palese, and A. Garcia-Sastre. 2005. Characterization of the reconstructed 1918 Spanish influenza pandemic virus. *Science* 310(5745):77-80.

U.S. Fish and Wildlife Service. 2007. *Nations with confirmed cases H5N1 avian influenza.* http://www.pandemicflu.gov/ (accessed July 27, 2007).

Woodward, T.E. 1994. *The Armed Forces Epidemiological Board: The histories of the commissions.* Washington, DC: Borden Institute, Office of the Surgeon General.

WHO (World Health Organization). 2005. *Avian influenza frequently asked questions.* http://www.who.int/csr/disease/avian_influenza/avian_faqs/en/index.html (accessed July 27, 2007).

WHO. 2007a. *H5N1 avian influenza: Timeline of major events*. http://www.who.int/csr/disease/avian_influenza/timeline_07_07_2007.pdf (accessed July 27, 2007).

WHO. 2007b. *Cumulative number of confirmed human cases of avian influenza A/(H5N1) reported to WHO*. http://www.who.int/csr/disease/avian_influenza/country/cases_table_2007_07_25/en/index.html (accessed July 27, 2007).

2

DoD-GEIS Headquarters AI/PI Management and Support Activities

In February 1999 the assistant secretary of defense for health affairs issued a memorandum outlining the operations of the Department of Defense's influenza surveillance activities. This memorandum directed the Department of Defense Global Emerging Infections Surveillance and Response System (DoD-GEIS) headquarters to provide professional guidance, direction, and oversight of DoD influenza surveillance efforts, with the U.S. Air Force as the lead agency for laboratory-based surveillance (Bailey, 1999). Between 1999 and 2005, DoD-GEIS headquarters coordinated a variety of DoD-conducted influenza surveillance activities at the Air Force Institute for Operational Health (AFIOH), the Naval Health Research Center (NHRC), and sites within the Military Health System (MHS) as well as the overseas laboratories. While DoD-GEIS headquarters directed a number of influenza projects, its primary role was as a funding source.[1]

On January 2, 2005, the 109th Congress passed H.R. 1815, Sec. 748, "Pandemic Avian Flu Preparedness," which listed DoD-GEIS by name and called upon the secretary of defense to address ". . . surveillance efforts domestically and internationally." Subsequently, the DoD-GEIS was tasked

[1]Institute of Medicine (IOM) Committee members visited DoD-GEIS headquarters in April 2007. Prior to this meeting DoD-GEIS headquarters provided the full committee with detailed background information on DoD-GEIS and the pandemic/avian influenza activities being supported by the headquarters. These materials were used in the writing of this chapter and are available from the IOM in the public access file.

by the assistant secretary of defense for health affairs to take the lead on the following activities laid out in Sec. 748, H.R. 1815:

- Surveillance efforts domestically and internationally, including those utilizing the Global Emerging Infections Systems (GEIS), and how such efforts are integrated with other ongoing surveillance systems
- Integration of pandemic and response planning with those of other federal departments, including the Department of Health and Human Services (HHS), Department of the Veterans Affairs, Department of State, and U.S. Agency for International Development
- Collaboration (as appropriate) with international entities engaged in pandemic preparedness and response

The supervisory role of DoD-GEIS headquarters in Avian Influenza/Pandemic Influenza (AI/PI) activities was further reinforced in 2006 when the U.S. Army Surgeon General designated DoD-GEIS as the oversight agency for the 2006 congressional AI/PI supplemental funding and as the responsible agency for "monitoring and reporting execution and outcomes . . . to improve pandemic and avian influenza surveillance for DoD" (Kiley, 2006).

In the fall of 2005, DoD-GEIS headquarters began to assess the gaps in DoD influenza surveillance and response activities in anticipation of the expansion of its influenza surveillance capability. The DoD-GEIS director submitted to the DoD-GEIS-supported laboratories and DoD agencies a December 22, 2005, memorandum, "Fiscal Year 2006 Special Supplemental Budget for Pandemic Influenza Preparedness," requesting the partners to submit surveillance proposals to carry out the mandate of the $39.28 million congressional supplemental appropriation that was soon to be distributed (Malone, 2005). In addition, DoD-GEIS headquarters worked closely with decision makers at the Office of the Assistant Secretary of Defense for Health Affairs, the Force Health Protection Council, the Army Executive Agency, and the Commander of U.S. Army Medical Research and Materiel Command to develop a strategy for handling the AI/PI funding and coordinate AI/PI activities across DoD.

Upon receipt of the AI/PI supplemental funds in March 2006, the recently appointed DoD-GEIS director reorganized the headquarters to create a separate influenza and zoonoses divisions, and, with the advice and consultation of the existing professional staff, the director developed an AI/PI emergency preparedness plan (AI/PI EPP) program concept of operations, outlining program priorities. In addition, the DoD-GEIS headquarters established a core staff of professional public health and scientific personnel to properly and responsibly execute these funds. The staff was to include an individual to serve as the leader of the supplemental influenza oversight team, and avian and pandemic emergency preparedness plan program, a communications center chief, a senior epidemiologist, an information systems analyst, a program manager, and a program assistant (see Box 2.1 for details on each position's role and responsibilities). Qualified candidates were sought, recruited, and interviewed with the assistance of the Henry M. Jackson Foundation (HJF)[2] human resources section, and they were hired during the subsequent six months. A total of nine positions were developed, six of which have been filled to date. To fill the three remaining positions, DoD-GEIS Headquarters would like to add a communications analyst, a junior epidemiologist, and a health education specialist to the staff. These additions are currently pending future funding and assessment of need for FY08.

DOD-GEIS AI/PI FUNDING

Because of the fiscal year 2006 supplemental funding, the AI/PI activities have become the largest component of the DoD-GEIS surveillance and response efforts. In fiscal year 2006, the total DoD-GEIS budget was $50.289 million, of which 78 percent—approximately $39 million—came from the fiscal year 2006 congressional supplemental for AI/PI. This represented a significant increase in DoD-GEIS funding from under $5 million in the program's first year of funding in fiscal year 1997 (see Figure 2.1).

At the time of this report 99.5 percent of the fiscal year 2006 supplemental funds had been obligated (see Table 2-1). The increase for fiscal year 2007 is also substantial though less, with a total estimated DoD-GEIS budget of $36.4 million, of which 69 percent, or $25 million, is expected to be AI/PI surveillance funding. All of these DoD-GEIS funds are directly appropriated from Defense Health Program dollars out of the Tricare Management Activity MHS.

While these AI/PI funds represent a substantial increase in the overall budget of DoD-GEIS in both fiscal year 2006 and fiscal year 2007, DoD-GEIS received less funding than was requested to carry out all of the proposed AI/PI activities. In fiscal year 2006, of $48 million requested, $39 million was approved. Similarly, in fiscal year 2007, of $50 million requested only $25 million was approved. Subsequently, in order to provide some consistency in influenza funding, a minimum level of funding was established, with a total of $40 million for fiscal year 2008 and $35 million for fiscal year 2009 being set during the DoD's early funding reviews, con-

[2]The Henry M. Jackson Foundation (HJF) for the Advancement of Military Medicine, Inc. is a private, not-for-profit organization dedicated to improving military medicine and public. HJF manages more than 60 endowments and 800 education funds that support military medical education and training (http://www.hjf.org/about/index.html).

BOX 2-1
DoD-GEIS Avian and Pandemic Influenza Emergency Preparedness Plan Program Staff's Role and Responsibilities

Team leader—provide direct scientific and medical support to the DoD-GEIS leadership; serve as epidemiology and public health subject matter expert for AI/PI related matters at DoD and other USG working groups and committees; provide technical and scientific consultative support to US military personnel and DoD officials; assist in the definition of relevant programmatic issues and decision-making process at the strategic, interagency, planning, and programmatic levels; assist DoD-GEIS management in the planning and direction, as well as improving the efficiency and effectiveness of, AI/PI activities; and prepare decision briefs, scientific manuscripts and presentations containing a variety of programmatic technical and funding information

Communications center chief—serve as the lead officer in charge of the communications center which will provide day-to-day support in information sharing activities with other DoD-GEIS partners and key stakeholders; responsible for the initial set-up and subsequent operation of all communications and information sharing capabilities; and directly responsible for the continuity of operation of the communications center and the day-to-day maintenance of electronic information

Senior epidemiologist—responsible for analyzing a variety of medical surveillance and field/lab epidemiologic data using statistical methods and computer hardware/software; draft research papers for peer-reviewed journals; assess the feasibility of proposed studies; evaluate data sources for other researchers; evaluate the suc-

ducted from October to December 2006. This permanent funding was coordinated and obtained on behalf of DoD-GEIS by the Office of the Assistant Secretary of Defense for Health Affairs (DoD-GEIS HQ, 2007a) through the inclusion of influenza funding in the program operation memorandum (POM) for the next two years.[3] It is still unclear if this POM status will be extended beyond 2009.

[3]The Program Objectives Memorandum (POM) is the annual estimating framework utilized by the Department of Defense. Department planning is then translated into programs/projects necessary to fulfill requirements and implement the plan. At the same time, cost estimates for requirements associated with said programs/projects are generated.

cess of policies and identify the need for other policies; provide assistance in the conduction of field epidemiologic and outbreak investigations; provide surveillance summaries and reports to the AI/PI program newsletter

Information systems analyst—plan, develop, test, and document highly complex applications programs. Generate new code and correct, convert, and/or modify existing code to meet specifications; confer with end-users to analyze specified methods and procedures, identify problems, and document specific requirements; Prepare reports on analyses, findings, and project progress, and present results to management and/or customer personnel; perform research on emerging technologies to determine impact on application execution

Program manager—Monitor and track costs, revenue, modifications, and billing for contracts performed by assigned office; compile and analyze complex contract, program, and financial data, and prepare monthly status reports based on the results; responsible for coordination of personnel travel, clearances, orders, set-up of video and teleconferences, and responsible for the administrative organization of DoD-GEIS sponsored meetings and symposia; serve as point of contact for the office on issues related to accounting, human resources, purchasing, and other departments, as well as external contacts such as customers, vendors, and subcontractors and security-related paperwork

Program assistant—responsible for travel requests, clearances, budgetary management and general office management support; collect and process purchasing requisitions, invoices for consultants and subcontractors, and travel and expense reports; provide work leadership to less experienced clerical and administrative personnel

HEADQUARTERS MANAGEMENT OF DOD-GEIS AI-PI ACTIVITIES

Based on the appropriations legislation and DoD directives mentioned above, DoD-GEIS headquarters is currently responsible for a variety of AI/PI tasks, including collaborating with U.S. and international AI/PI partners, disseminating information and data generated by DoD-GEIS AI/PI activities, and overseeing and providing support to AI/PI projects run by the domestic and overseas laboratories and other DoD facilities. Thus the majority of the DoD-GEIS headquarters AI/PI supplemental funds ($1,634,100) are dedicated to managing multi-service DoD AI/PI programs and ensuring that available resources are utilized rapidly and effectively. In order to achieve this goal, DoD-GEIS headquarters has established an AI/PI EPP Management Office and Communications Center and created a cadre of dedicated personnel in AI/PI matters to enable the effective administration of a $30-40 million/year program. The establishment of management centers and the

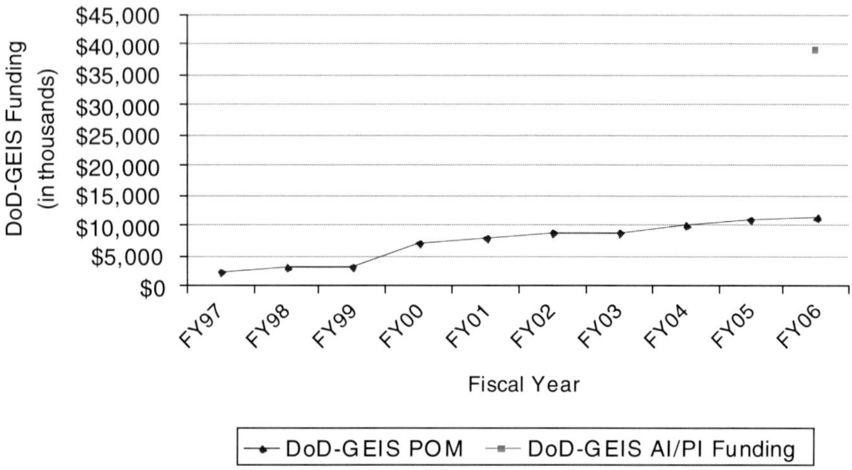

FIGURE 2-1 DoD-GEIS funding from fiscal year 1997 to 2006.
SOURCE: DoD-GEIS HQ, 2007b.

TABLE 2-1 DoD-GEIS Avian Influenza/Pandemic Influenza Supplemental Funding in Fiscal Year 2006

Organization Funded	Dollar Amount Approved (in thousands)	Dollar Amount Obligated (in thousands)	Percent Obligated
DoD-GEIS HQ	$5,447	$5,447	100.0%
NAMRU-2	$2,665	$2,622	98.4%
AFRIMS	$6,140	$6,110	99.5%
NAMRU-3	$3,988	$3,986	99.9%
USAMRU-K	$2,634	$2,634	100.0%
NMRCD	$1,741	$1,741	100.0%
NHRC	$3,164	$3,164	100.0%
AFIOH	$4,182	$4,182	100.0%
Other Organizations[a]	$9,084	$8,967	98.7%
Total	$39,045	$38,853	99.5%

[a]"Other Organizations" include USAMRIID ($394,000), LRMC (Germany) ($835,000), 18th MEDCOM (Korea) ($89,000), AFIP ($63,000), BAMC ($117,000), CDHAM/USUHS ($263,000), USACHPPM ($3,347,000), VETCOM ($15,000), PACAF ($45,000), NEHC ($954,000), NEPMU-5 ($14,000), WRAIR (PM Div) ($1,940,000), and ASD(HA)-FHP&R ($900,000).
SOURCE: DoD-GEIS, 2007b.

expansion of relevant staff has increased the ability of DoD-GEIS headquarters to collaborate with relevant partners, communicate vital information to other DoD facilities as well as to national and global organizations, and oversee and manage the AI/PI projects being conducted at all DoD domestic and overseas laboratories (DoD-GEIS HQ, 2007a).

Oversight and Management

Although the DoD-GEIS headquarters has no command or control over the assets and personnel of any of the DoD-GEIS-supported laboratories or DoD agencies, DoD-GEIS uses influence derived from its centralized control of AI/PI activities funding and close coordination with the office of the assistant secretary of defense for health affairs to oversee and manage a large program across multiple commands (see Figure 2.2).

DoD-GEIS headquarters staff guided the establishment and development of influenza and AI/PI surveillance and response activities. In addition, the staffs of the influenza and zoonoses division and the epidemiology and health systems division have had ample opportunity to interact with DoD-GEIS-supported laboratories and DoD agencies in addressing program priorities and problems by exchange of information, provision of guidance, and periodic telephone conferences and site visits. The principal activities and functions of the DoD-GEIS headquarters staff in support of AI/PI surveillance and response activities are as follows (DoD-GEIS HQ, 2007a):

(1) Provide scientific and administrative oversight of DoD influenza surveillance efforts as well as of AI/PI EPP program initiatives to include, but not limited to, the following:

(a) Initial development and scientific, merit-based evaluation of AI/PI control program-related surveillance and research proposals

(b) Establishment of monitoring guidelines and formats for routine, periodic monthly status situation reports and status reports on AI/PI control program-related proposals

(c) Centralized management of budgetary and contract management activities

(d) Coordination of facilities infrastructure, maintenance and other program management activities with supporting agencies such as the HJF

(2) Provide centralized subject matter expertise to DoD-GEIS partners in the areas of influenza and other acute respiratory infection (ARI) and AI/PI control.

(3) Establish and maintain a central communications center capability for coordination of influenza and other ARIs and AI/PI EPP program and other DoD-GEIS activities with special emphasis toward key information

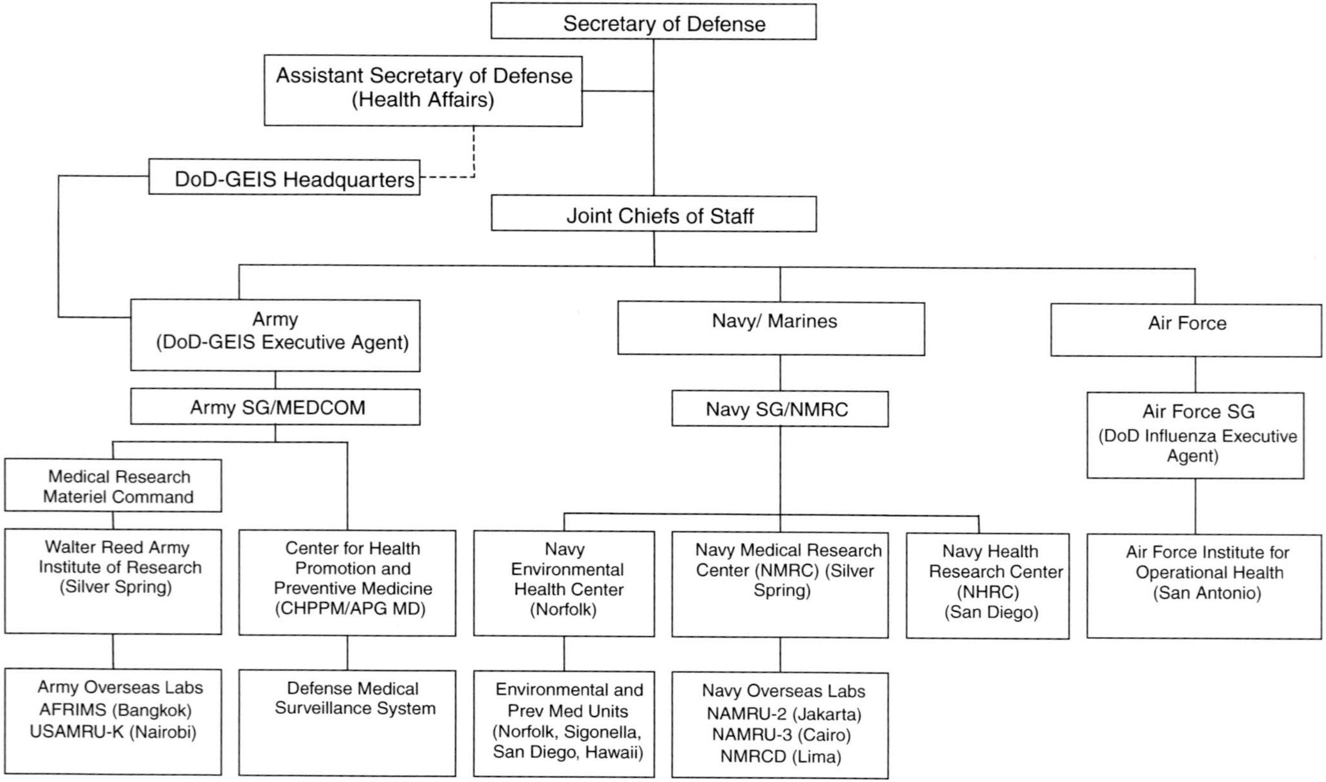

FIGURE 2-2 DoD-GEIS organizational chart.

and updates on DoD AI/PI EPP program-related activities in strategic areas of the world.

(4) Provide specialized AI/PI EPP-related epidemiological, laboratory, and communications expertise in support of exercises and real-time outbreaks of influenza or other emerging infectious diseases (EIDs) in coordination with the office of the assistant secretary of defense for health affairs, the Office of the Army Surgeon General, the Naval Bureau of Medicine and Surgery, the Air Force Surgeon General's office, and the Combatant Command (COCOM) surgeons' offices.

(5) Assist in the development and facilitation of tabletop emergency-preparedness exercises as well as in the support of ongoing medical training and education activities in AI/PI control program-related matters in coordination with the Uniformed Services University of the Health Sciences (USUHS), COCOM surgeons, and other DoD-GEIS partners.

(6) Provide an integrated and standardized methodology for clinical laboratory testing of patient samples suspected of infection with influenza and other militarily relevant EIDs, consistent with the World Health Organization (WHO) and the Centers for Disease Control and Prevention (CDC) systems in coordination with DoD influenza reference centers in the United States (AFIOH and NHRC) as well as with the respective services clinical laboratory consultants and major medical centers.

DoD-GEIS headquarters staff maintains constant supervision and oversight of AI/PI efforts through review and feedback in monthly reports submitted to the AI/PI EPP program staff, which includes statements of performance and status of funding obligations by each partner. Metrics reviewed within these monthly reports include, but are not limited to, the number of specimens collected and processed, the number of sites participating in isolate collection, the number of countries participating in isolate collection, and the number of Biosafety Level 3 (BSL-3) labs completed and functioning (DoD-GEIS HQ, 2007a). Constant feedback is being provided when deficiencies are identified, and subsequent funding—provided on a quarterly basis—is contingent on progress made by DOD-GEIS-supported laboratories and DoD agencies. AI/PI supplemental funding obligations are monitored centrally, and subsequent allocation of funding is adjusted based on performance—or lack thereof. Based on these measures, DoD-GEIS headquarters sees the execution of the fiscal year 2006 congressional supplement for AI/PI, the efficient obligation of funds, and the accomplishment of project goals by the DoD-GEIS headquarters staff and DOD-GEIS-supported laboratories and DoD agencies (99.5 percent obligation of fiscal year 2006 funds) as positive indications of the program's capacity for utilization of limited, one-year funding.

An additional component of oversight and management is the provision of influenza-related guidance, mentoring, and analytic support to entities executing the DoD-GEIS AI/PI program. DoD-GEIS headquarters currently relies on information sharing and posting of data and key event information within the GEIS website as part of the communications center functions (DoD-GEIS HQ, 2007a). Mentoring is conducted on a project-by-project basis; input and comments are provided on project execution. Data collection, analysis, and assistance are provided in final write-ups of project results for publication or presentation. Joint meetings to present project updates and to discuss future directions are held periodically, such as the DoD Joint Influenza Surveillance Working Group held annually in May, the Force Health Protection Conference held annually in August, the International Conference on Emerging Infectious Diseases held every other March, and the State of the DoD-GEIS meeting, which was held most recently in December 2005. In addition, DoD-GEIS headquarters staff make periodic visits to the overseas laboratories and other working partners at least twice a year to discuss priorities and plan future activities. Best products and practices are also shared between DoD-GEIS partners, such as the transplantation of the Early Warning Outbreak Recognition System (EWORS) from the Naval Medical Research Unit No.2 (NAMRU-2) in Indonesia to the Naval Medical Research Center in Peru (DoD-GEIS HQ, 2007a). Expertise is also transferred between laboratories as a result of medical scientist career management by the Army and Navy; personnel are often reassigned from one DoD-GEIS partner to another, providing additional "cross fertilization." The DoD-GEIS headquarters seeks to maximize the analytic capacities and expertise within the DoD-GEIS network to assist DoD-GEIS-supported laboratories and DoD agencies instead of developing separate and independent analytic activities or resources. Limited technical assistance is provided to certain projects by drawing on the epidemiology and data analysis resources at the U.S. Army's Medical Surveillance Activity co-located with DoD-GEIS headquarters at the Linden Lane location in Silver Spring, Md. (DoD-GEIS HQ, 2007a).

Collaboration

DoD-GEIS is working to coordinate and integrate its efforts with national and international surveillance and response-planning partners, such as CDC, HHS, the Pan American Health Organization (PAHO), WHO, and the U.S. Department of Agriculture's Animal and Plant Health Inspection Service.

DoD-GEIS staff participates in a number of DoD-run influenza collaborating bodies, including annual DoD Joint Influenza Surveillance Working Group meetings (Embrey, 2006). This meeting is typically sponsored by

NHRC or AFIOH and brings together domestic and international influenza-surveillance efforts from within DoD. While this primarily involves DoD working groups, non-DoD agencies such as the CDC and the U.S. Agency for International Development also participate. During these meetings the various organizations share surveillance data and identify potential surveillance gaps that can be and need to be addressed. Additionally, DoD-GEIS headquarters staff hosts a biweekly teleconference with service epidemiology centers and key partners to exchange timely information on infectious threats to U.S. forces and to coordinate outbreak response; it is referred to as the EpiChiefs Teleconference. Participants include the Navy Environmental Health Center, the U.S. Army Center for Health Promotion and Preventive Medicine, the Armed Forces Institute of Pathology, the U.S. Northern Command, and the Assistant Secretary of Defense for Health Affairs, among others (DoD-GEIS HQ, 2007a).

DoD-GEIS staff also participate in two HHS-coordinated influenza-related groups. The first is a quarterly meeting with both the influenza division and the Office of Global Health at HHS. DoD-GEIS's participation in this group allows for ongoing feedback regarding influenza and AI/PI surveillance and control activities. These meetings focus upon the identification and evaluation of potential gaps in surveillance efforts in an effort minimize duplication as well as on the review of spending plans related to pandemic influenza activities. Another purpose of these meetings is to enhance surveillance capabilities and the reporting of timely information through coordination and cooperation between the two organizations. DoD-GEIS was designated by the Assistant Secretary of Defense for Health Affairs as the DoD point of contact and the meeting coordinator for this endeavor.

DoD-GEIS and representatives from other DoD Offices are also members of the HHS Pandemic and Seasonal Influenza Risk Management Group. This group has met monthly since its creation in September 2006. Representatives from HHS, the National Institutes of Health (NIH), the U.S. Department of Agriculture, the Food and Drug Administration (FDA), the State Department, and CDC participate in this meeting and its related topic-driven focus area groups. Surveillance of pandemic influenza is one of the many focus areas of this group, along with research and development, animal models, manufacturing capacity, regulatory and legal issues, and stockpile issues. Currently two of the three working groups, vaccine prioritization and influenza diagnostics, have DoD representation (DoD-GEIS HQ, 2007a).

DoD representatives also collaborate with many of these same partners at the annual meetings of the FDA-sponsored Vaccines and Related Biological Products Advisory Committee. This advisory committee meets once a year to discuss the globally circulating strains of influenza viruses in an attempt to decide which strains to include in the annual seasonal influenza vaccine administered in the Northern Hemisphere. At this meeting, DoD-GEIS presents annual influenza surveillance data collected through its related activities. Representatives from the FDA, HHS, NIH, academia, and vaccine manufacturers also attend this meeting and make presentations (DoD-GEIS HQ, 2007a).

In addition to formalized working groups, DoD and other government agencies, including HHS, the Department of Homeland Security (DHS), the State Department, and CDC, have exchanged full-time medical liaison officers to help provide situational awareness of ongoing missions and to implement initiatives of mutual interest (Bresee and Jernigan, 2006). Professional relationships with key individuals in these organizations provide DoD-GEIS staff with unique and invaluable opportunities to seek, share, and receive advice about incorporating best methods and practices. DoD-GEIS also has considerable ongoing professional contact with senior scientists and program managers from other federal agencies through its regular participation with, and membership in, major activities such as the Institute of Medicine's Microbial Threat Forum, the U.S. Medicine Institute's roundtable policy meetings, and the Infectious Diseases Society of America.

External advice and consultation for AI/PI surveillance and control activities is received on a project-by-project basis from outside consultants such as key offices at PAHO, WHO, and the Food and Agricultural Organization. The assignment of a full-time U.S. military medical officer to WHO in Geneva, Switzerland, has bolstered coordination and integration of efforts between DoD-GEIS and WHO (Fukuda, 2006).

DoD-GEIS has also used the supplemental funding to create and fund a number of coordinating mechanisms and events related to AI/PI, including

- development of DoD-GEIS biweekly EpiChiefs and other ad hoc executive summary reports distributed to key DoD military and civilian health officials;
- development of training efforts and coordinating AI/PI preparedness workshops in support of five combatant commands in conjunction with the USUHS Center for Disaster and Humanitarian Assistance officials; and
- oversight and coordination of the CDC-DoD Working Group on Influenza and Emerging Infectious Diseases, which AI-PI EPP program office staff assumed in October 2006 (DoD-GEIS HQ, 2007a).

Communication

The DoD-GEIS headquarters communications center, established in October 2006, is the centerpiece of DoD-GEIS' communication strategy. The DOD-GEIS headquarters is now able to quickly distribute information and disease updates to its various partners and key stakeholders via an electronic forum. Information is gathered through open sources and regular communication channels and then widely disseminated. Although many recipients of this material are DoD personnel, other government agencies are included, such as the State Department, DHS, CDC, HHS, and the Office of the Vice President, in addition to the international WHO and PAHO. Currently, 139 individuals representing key offices from seven U.S. government agencies, various international health organizations, and many DoD health commands receive information on a daily basis regarding infectious diseases (primarily influenza), surveillance updates, and new disease outbreaks (DoD-GEIS HQ, 2007a).

DoD-GEIS headquarters and the AI/PI surveillance and response efforts office have recently relocated, and a functional DoD-GEIS communications center has been established on-site with video teleconferencing and telecom capabilities and a DoD-GEIS communication center e-mail resource for the centralized distribution of information to the director of DoD-GEIS, the Assistant Secretary of Defense for Health Affairs, and other relevant service components and government partners, such as the CDC and DHHS as it becomes available. The communications center is also capable of providing 24 hours a day, seven days a week communications between all DoD-GEIS partners during a pandemic if the DoD determined this action necessary. The DoD-GEIS communications center complements the outreach and reporting role of AFIOH and other organizations within DoD that perform critical influenza surveillance, such as NHRC and the U.S. Army Center for Health Promotion and Preventive Medicine-Europe. In an emergency pandemic influenza situation, the communications center will be available for operations 24 hours a day, seven days a week and will coordinate all communications dealing with influenza surveillance and response provided by DoD-GEIS partners (DoD-GEIS HQ, 2007a). In addition to the new office space and the communications center, DoD-GEIS headquarters has plans to initiate an AI/PI EPP Program Management Office which will provide overall management and oversight of the routine ARI surveillance and newly developed AI/PI-related surveillance projects at the DoD-GEIS.

The key stakeholders with whom the headquarters communicates include, but are not limited to, the following (DoD-GEIS HQ, 2007a):

a. The Office of the Assistant Secretary of Defense for Health Affairs
b. Surgeons General for the U.S. Army, U.S. Navy and U.S. Air Force
c. Unified Combatant Command surgeons' offices;
d. U.S. military medical treatment facilities in the United States and overseas
e. Domestic U.S. military medical reference laboratories (AFIOH, NHRC)
f. International reference laboratories for influenza (such as specific offices at DHS, WHO, and the CDC)
g. DoD overseas medical research laboratories
h. The U.S. Army Center for Health Promotion and Preventive Medicine
i. The Armed Forces Medical Intelligence Center
j. The DHS's National Biosurveillance Integration Center
k. The U.S. Army Medical Research and Materiel Command and applicable associated activities (such as the Walter Reed Army Institute of Research and NMRC)

One of the objectives of this communications center is to be a central, single source of accurate, timely information on global influenza for stakeholders within various U.S. government agencies. Documents that are disseminated are subsequently posted on the DoD-GEIS website, either on the public or the secure site, depending on the level of sensitivity of the information. DoD-GEIS partners regularly report on outbreaks occurring within their host countries and regions. Laboratory confirmation of the presence of novel viruses (e.g., H5N1) is also considered a priority communication to DoD-GEIS headquarters from the field.

DOD-GEIS HEADQUARTERS AND OTHER MILITARY HEALTH SYSTEM INFLUENZA SURVEILLANCE AND RESPONSE ACTIVITIES

DoD-GEIS Headquarters Influenza Activities

In addition to managing projects being carried out by other DoD partners, DoD-GEIS headquarters works directly with the Johns Hopkins University Applied Physics Laboratory (JHU/APL) to manage and execute several influenza-related projects. Two of these projects funded with AI/PI supplemental funding are an evaluation of the Early Warning Surveillance/

BOX 2-2
Early Warning Outbreak Recognition System (EWORS)

The Early Warning Outbreak Recognition System (EWORS) was developed by NAMRU-2 to detect disease outbreaks early throughout Indonesia without relying on slower and often nonexistent laboratory methods. EWORS is based on a simple computer program that allows a remote clinic to enter basic demographic data on the patient and document whether they have symptoms such as fever, diarrhea, breathing difficulty, cough, or vomiting. These data are downloaded daily from remote sites around the country to a central location such as the ministry of health. Either remotely or locally, data can then be graphed based on variables such as date, age, race, and symptoms and presented geographically by area of residence to determine clustering by location. It is now also being used in Peru as well to collect surveillance data on a symptoms associate with influenza.

Response System (EWORS) and an expansion of the Pandemic Influenza Policy Model (PIPM).

Early Warning Surveillance/Response System Strengthening

DoD-GEIS headquarters is using $460,000 in fiscal year 2006 AI/PI supplemental funding to strengthen DoD-GEIS's existing EWORS system (see Box 2-2). In collaborating with overseas DoD-GEIS partners, such as DoD overseas laboratories, DoD-GEIS will use the surveillance/response system evaluation framework, results from the modeling/simulation studies, and field evaluations (all conducted with supplemental funds) to implement early warning surveillance/response systems targeted for pandemic influenza but applicable to other emerging infections as well.

The seven-person team at JHU/APL working on this project draws heavily on collaborations with NAMRU-2 in Jakarta and NMRCD in Lima, both of which have developed electronic syndromic surveillance systems with host-country ministries of health with previous funding from DoD-GEIS and other agencies. DoD-GEIS headquarters hopes to pilot the next-generation EWORS system using data gained during this project, including a comprehensive evaluation of existing EWORS systems. Key EWORS staff members from NAMRU-2 and NMRCD participate in an ongoing working group with JHU/APL and DoD-GEIS headquarters staff to guide enhancement of existing EWORS networks and planning for new systems (DoD-GEIS HQ, 2007a). DoD-GEIS anticipates that this AI/PI-funded project will greatly enhance existing EWORS systems and will guide future investment by DoD-GEIS and other agencies and governments in early warning systems in resource-poor countries.

Pandemic Influenza Policy Model Expansion

DoD-GEIS headquarters is also supporting the expansion of the Pandemic Influenza Policy Model with $460,000 in supplemental funding. PIPM is a modeling project initiated to provide information on influenza preparedness to military installations in order to allow them to plan for various pandemic scenarios. The expansion of the PIPM is expected to provide the means to examine the effect of changing disease and operational parameters on a wider range of DoD installations and organizations, including basic-training installations of the U.S. Navy and U.S. Air Force, installations with high operational tempo, installations with high logistical throughput, installations undergoing large-scale mobilization or demobilization operations, and installations within large metropolitan areas. Methods will be applied from operations research theory, including linear and dynamic programming along with other optimization techniques as applicable, to expand the PIPM model. In addition, the expanded PIPM model will incorporate and expand aspects of existing models, such as CDC's FluAid and FluSurge and DoD's Joint Medical Planning software, in order to address requirements that are unique to the military (DoD-GEIS HQ, 2007a).

DoD-GEIS and the project team from JHU/APL have divided the work into three phases. In the first phase, data will be collected on a variety of types of military installations to understand how the PIPM needs to be expanded to accommodate the inclusion of those installations in the model. Then the project team will focus on identification and prioritization of pertinent disease and operational parameters that will affect the DoD medical response to pandemic influenza. In the second phase, information gathered from the various sources will be collated, and estimated DoD-specific values for the parameters will be identified. The project team will also construct and evaluate a decision-analysis model that optimizes DoD public health response to pandemic influenza. In the last phase, the web-based and user-friendly PIPM computer interface will be extended to allow DoD personnel to plan for, evaluate, and train on different disease scenarios for a wide range of military installations and organizations (DoD-GEIS HQ, 2007a). DoD-GEIS headquarters expects that this project will provide military medical and operational commanders and policy makers with the first fine-grained, military-specific simulation tool for testing pandemic influenza surveillance and response strategies. Given that the 1918 pandemic severely affected military populations, the ability to evaluate preparedness and preventive measures against a H5N1 pandemic model is seen as important.

Influenza Activities Elsewhere in the Military Health System

United States Army Medical Research Institute of Infectious Diseases

In fiscal year 2006, GEIS supplemental funding for pandemic and avian influenza was the only source of funding for work done at the U.S. Army Medical Research Institute of Infectious Diseases with highly pathogenic avian influenza (DoD-GEIS, 2007). The institute conducted a number of activities supported by supplemental influenza funds, including analysis of influenza molecular diagnostics, generation of an influenza A reference panel, and development of immunodiagnostic reagents for influenza diagnosis (DoD-GEIS, 2007). To support the influenza activities, the institute purchased specialized equipment for highly pathogenic avian influenza work, and personnel were trained in biosafety practices. As a result, the institute now provides DoD and GEIS with a unique high-containment laboratory capable of supporting work with highly pathogenic avian influenza (DoD-GEIS, 2007).

United States Army Center for Health Promotion and Preventive Medicine

Serosurveillance for avian and pandemic influenza In fiscal year 2006, work was initiated to develop a Center for Epidemiology and Serosurveillance of Pandemic Influenza associated with the DoD Serum Repository. The primary objectives of this center were to be assessing the prevalence of exposure to avian influenza strains among military service members, providing serologic data to support investigations of geographically localized avian and pandemic influenza outbreaks, and investigating the prevalence of a preexisting antibody against human influenza strains that may provide the potential for cross-reactive protection from avian influenza infection among service members in the event of an avian and pandemic influenza outbreak. The supplemental influenza funding was used to support the development of this center. Additional staff were hired to implement and oversee the project. Detailed programs were generated to identify service members deployed to or living in areas of H5N1 activity through the Defense Medical Surveillance System. The Southern Research Institute in Birmingham, Ala., was selected to perform both avian (H5N1 clades 1 and 2 subtypes) and human influenza (H3N2 and H1N1) seroprevalence testing on DoD serum repository specimens, using hemagglutination inhibition assays with confirmatory microneutralization assays. Specimen testing began early in 2007. The U.S. Army Center for Health Promotion and Preventive Medicine expects that this work will provide a unique opportunity to generate seroepidemiologic data to enable surveillance for H5N1 and related avian and pandemic influenza virus exposure and to permit rational vaccine or therapeutic selection in the event of an outbreak.

Pandemic Influenza Workshop On August 7-8, 2006, the U.S. Army Center for Health Promotion and Preventive Medicine and DoD-GEIS headquarters sponsored a training course aimed at improving preparedness and response to an influenza pandemic. The workshop, held in Albuquerque, N. Mex., was supported by the supplemental funding for pandemic and avian influenza. The target audience comprised military public health emergency officers and other public health practitioners. More than 300 participants from the Army, Navy, Air Force, Marines, and Coast Guard participated, as well as personnel from other U.S. government agencies, including the Departments of Veterans Affairs and Homeland Security, and also from the militaries of allied countries. The workshop covered lessons learned from previous pandemics and the swine influenza response in 1976, surveillance for influenza and emerging pathogens, and components of the national, DoD, COCOM, and U.S. Army Medical Command efforts toward preparedness. Other areas were also discussed, including community preparedness, incident command at the local level, pharmacological and nonpharmacological methods of preventing and slowing the spread of infection, triage and treatment options, use of personal protective equipment, legal considerations involved in responding to a pandemic, communications during a pandemic, and the management of mass fatalities.

CONCLUSIONS

The committee has found that given condensed time frames for planning and implementation, DoD-GEIS has effectively executed and managed the fiscal year 2006 AI/PI supplemental funding. The DoD-GEIS headquarters has facilitated the disbursement and utilization of the large increase in funding to influenza programs, building both DoD and host-country laboratory and human resources capacity. It has expanded the information being collected about avian influenza and acute respiratory diseases and has strengthened U.S. relations with the global community. DoD-GEIS headquarters has successfully managed the implementation of these AI/PI projects through the following activities: the addition of project management staff as well as the increase in relevant influenza surveillance and response expertise; the establishment of assessment mechanisms to track the progress of AI/PI projects; their participation in U.S. government working groups on influenza preparedness and response; and the establishment of the inter-DoD communication center to facilitate the sharing of influenza information across laboratory facilities.

While the committee concludes that the execution of the fiscal year

2006 AI/PI supplemental funding has resulted in the implementation of valuable influenza surveillance and response activities and that the changes to DoD-GEIS headquarters have contributed to improvements to the DoD-GEIS influenza programs, there are a number of areas that should be strengthened in order to improve a sustained DoD-GEIS influenza surveillance and response effort.

First, the AI/PI supplemental funding and the associated DoD directives have led to strengthening the role of DoD-GEIS headquarters as the responsible agency for coordination, guidance, and oversight of DoD influenza activities. The committee has concluded that a strengthening of this leadership role in conjunction with a reexamination and revision of the functional operating structure of the DoD influenza and respiratory disease surveillance program to reflect the current needs of the program would improve the management and oversight of the program in general.

> **RECOMMENDATION 2-1. In order to better manage the influenza program, DoD-GEIS headquarters should strengthen its leadership role in the execution of DoD-GEIS influenza activities through strategic planning and distribution of future funding.**

Second, while there have been attempts to improve inter-laboratory dialogue and information sharing, laboratories are still working in varying degrees of isolation and would benefit from closer collaboration. Since the laboratories are relatively new to the influenza field, many of them have experienced a steep learning curve over the past fiscal year. Each laboratory has gained valuable lessons from implementing the first year of these supplemental AI/PI funds, and this knowledge, if shared, would greatly improve the continued program development of AI/PI activities at all DoD-GEIS sites. Thus, in order to most effectively improve DoD-GEIS's influenza activities, there should be strategic planning done at DOD-GEIS headquarters based on lessons learned at the laboratories over the first year of supplemental funding.

> **RECOMMENDATION 2-2. In order to assure the most effective use of the resources and varied expertise at the different DoD sites, mechanisms should be put into place to have systematic communication among the sites with respect to the various influenza-related projects and activities, including the development of a structured communication mechanism within each laboratory that would interact with headquarters to coordinate influenza activities, and the creation of regular opportunities for sharing of best practices facilitated by DoD-GEIS headquarters.**

Third, the committee concluded that the addition of relevant expertise at DoD-GEIS headquarters was benefiting the whole DoD-GEIS influenza program. Plans to further strengthen the headquarters personnel would allow DoD-GEIS headquarters to more appropriately address the issues and challenges faced at the DoD-GEIS-supported laboratories. For example, DoD-GEIS headquarters is planning to add a communications analyst, a junior epidemiologist, and a health education specialist to the staff. These additions are currently pending future funding and assessment of need in fiscal year 2008.

RECOMMENDATION 2-3. In order to improve the management of the DoD-GEIS influenza program, DoD-GEIS headquarters should continue to strengthen its in-house influenza expertise as necessary in order to give DoD laboratories and other relevant institutions the assistance needed to implement quality influenza surveillance and response activities.

Finally, collaboration and coordination between DoD-GEIS and other partners helps to limit redundancies and to maximize resources for AI/PI activities. It is important that one of the primary occupations of the headquarters be the active coordination and guidance of projects carried out across all DoD-GEIS-funded facilities with those activities being conducted by other U.S. agencies and international partners.

RECOMMENDATION 2-4. DoD-GEIS headquarters should continue to work with U.S. and international partners to ensure coordination among global influenza efforts.

REFERENCES

Bailey, S. 1999. Policy for DoD global, laboratory-based influenza surveillance. *Memorandum for Surgeon General of the Army, Surgeon General of the Navy, Surgeon General of the Air Force, Deputy Director for Medical Readiness, J-4, the Joint Staff.* U.S. Department of Defense, Health Affairs, Washington, DC, February 3, 1999. On file with the National Academies Public Access Records Office.

Bresee, J., and D. Jernigan. 2006. *U.S. government contributions to global influenza surveillance.* PowerPoint presentation given at first meeting of the IOM Committee for the Assessment of DoD-GEIS Influenza Surveillance and Response Programs, December 19, Washington, DC.

DoD-GEIS (Department of Defense-Global Emerging Infections System). 2007. *Partnering in the fight against emerging infections: Annual report, fiscal year 2006.* Silver Spring, MD: Walter Reed Army Institute for Research

DoD-GEIS HQ. 2007a. *Presentation on DoD-GEIS headquarters activities.* Presented April 30, 2007 at DoD-GEIS Headquarters in Silver Spring, MD.

DoD-GEIS HQ. 2007b. *DoD-GEIS funding distribution to all GEIS partners from fiscal year 1997 to 2006* (unpublished).

Embrey, E. P. 2006. *U.S. government policy perspectives on global influenza.* PowerPoint presentation given at first meeting of the IOM Committee for the Assessment of DoD-GEIS Influenza Surveillance and Response Programs, December 19, Washington, DC.

Kiley, K. 2006. *Oversight for supplemental funding for pandemic and avian influenza memorandum.* Memorandum for Surgeon General of the Army, Surgeon General of the Navy, Surgeon General of the Air Force. Signed March 16, 2006.

Fukuda, K. 2006. *Global challenges of pandemic and avian influenza.* PowerPoint presentation given at first meeting of the IOM Committee for the Assessment of DoD-GEIS Influenza Surveillance and Response Programs, December 19, Washington, D.C.

Malone, J. L. 2005. *Fiscal year 2006 special supplemental budget for pandemic influenza preparedness memorandum.* Memorandum for DoD-GEIS-supported laboratories and DoD agencies. December 22, 2005.

LIST OF CONTACTS

LT Jean-Paul Chretien, Coordinator, Overseas Research Laboratories, Department of Defense Global Emerging Infections Surveillance and Response System headquarters

Mario DaRocha, Program Assistant, Department of Defense Global Emerging Infections Surveillance and Response System headquarters

Dr. Tracy DuVernoy, Chief, Communications Center, Department of Defense Global Emerging Infections Surveillance and Response System headquarters

COL Ralph Erickson, Director, Department of Defense Global Emerging Infections Surveillance and Response System headquarters

Dr. Joel Gaydos, Public Health Practice, Department of Defense Global Emerging Infections Surveillance and Response System headquarters

Steve Gubenia, Deputy, Finance and Administration, Department of Defense Global Emerging Infections Surveillance and Response System headquarters

LtCol Victor MacIntosh, Director, Military Health System GEIS Programs, Department of Defense Global Emerging Infections Surveillance and Response System headquarters

Jay Mansfield, Information Systems Analyst/Programmer, Department of Defense Global Emerging Infections Surveillance and Response System headquarters

Robin Miliner, Program Manager, Department of Defense Global Emerging Infections Surveillance and Response System headquarters

Dr. Jean Otto, Senior Epidemiologist, Department of Defense Global Emerging Infections Surveillance and Response System headquarters

Dr. Jose Sanchez, Leader, Influenza Team, Department of Defense Global Emerging Infections Surveillance and Response System headquarters

LTC Kelly Vest, Deputy Influenza and Zoonoses, Department of Defense Global Emerging Infections Surveillance and Response System headquarters

Col Mark Rubertone, Chief, Army Medical Surveillance Activity

Dr. Angelia Eick, Deputy Scientific Director, Center for Biosurveillance, Army Medical Surveillance Activity

3

Naval Medical Research Unit 2 Indonesia Avian and Pandemic Influenza Activities

The Naval Medical Research Unit No. 2 (NAMRU-2), originally established during World War II in Guam and later relocated, first to Taiwan and then to the Philippines, began operating a detachment in Jakarta, Indonesia, in 1970. Its mission at that point was to investigate infectious diseases of military importance both for the U.S. Navy and for the rest of the Department of Defense (DoD) (DoD-GEIS, 2007a). It has recently played a very important role in the surveillance of avian influenza and a potential pandemic (see Figure 3-1).

Historically NAMRU-2 has focused on applied research in support of its medical mission. Its past research activities provided a strong foundation for the expanded focus of the DoD's Global Emerging Infections Surveillance and Response System (DoD-GEIS) on surveillance and response capacity. Avian influenza highlights the issues of regional disease spread and also the significant role that NAMRU-2 plays in conducting disease surveillance, case and outbreak investigation, and diagnostic support. NAMRU-2 either identified or shared in the confirmation of all recent human cases of H5N1 infection in Indonesia, where the laboratory is recognized as one of two H5N1 reference laboratories by the Ministry of Health (MoH).

A site visit team of the Institute of Medicine (IOM) Committee for the Assessment of Department of Defense Global Emerging Infections Surveillance and Response System visited NAMRU-2 from March 4-10, 2006.[1]

[1]Prior to the NAMRU-2 visit, the laboratory staff provided the committee with detailed background information on NAMRU-2 and the pandemic/avian influenza activities it was supporting. These materials are available from the IOM in the Public Access File.

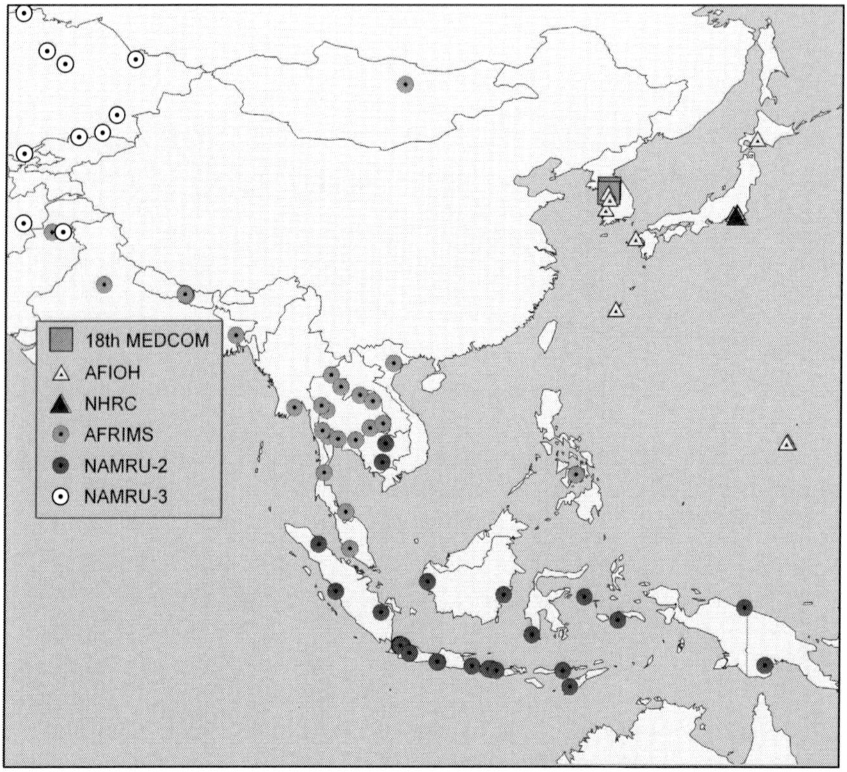

FIGURE 3-1 DoD's regional presence in influenza surveillance (South East Asia), 2007.
SOURCE: DoD-GEIS, 2007b.

During the team's visit, its members also toured a NAMRU-2 extension facility in Phnom Penh, Cambodia. A list of the people that the team met and interviewed along with the itinerary that the team followed can be found at the end of this chapter.

INFLUENZA IN INDONESIA

Indonesia, home to 224 million people and 1.3 billion poultry, including 920 million chickens and 48 million ducks, reported its first human case of H5N1 avian influenza in July 2005 (Naipospos, 2007; WHO, 2007a). Since then it has experienced more avian flu fatalities than any other country in the world, with its 97th case confirmed in late May 2007 (WHO, 2007a).

In addition to Indonesia having the highest number of H5N1 AI cases worldwide, it has also experienced the largest family cluster of confirmed cases. In May 2006, seven human cases were reported in the Karo district of North Sumatra, all of whom were close relatives of the suspected initial case. Though the disease did not spread beyond the extended family, limited human-to-human transmission of the virus was not entirely ruled out. Full genetic sequencing of viruses isolated from cases in this cluster found no evidence of genetic reassortment or significant mutations, and subsequent outbreak clusters in Indonesia also failed to provide evidence of human-to-human transmission (WHO, 2006a; WHO, 2007a).

In addition to Indonesia, eight countries in Southeast Asia have reported highly pathogenic avian influenza among poultry, namely Bangladesh, Cambodia, India, Laos, Malaysia, Myanmar, Thailand, and Vietnam. Both Bangladesh and Myanmar reported outbreaks of highly pathogenic H5N1 in poultry in early 2007. Indonesia reported its first human case of H5N1 avian influenza in July 2005 (WHO, 2007a; WHO, 2007b).

MANAGEMENT AND PLANNING

Staffing

DoD-GEIS projects at NAMRU-2 are overseen by the laboratory science director. At the time of the IOM visit by the site team, NAMRU-2 staff included 21 Americans. In addition, NAMRU-2 employs a staff of more than 120 foreign service nationals (FSNs). FSN staff includes laboratory technicians and contract support personnel with expertise in areas of management and administration. All department heads have significant involvement in programs other than DoD-GEIS and avian influenza/pandemic influenza (AI/PI) activities, including Military Infectious Diseases Research Program (MIDRP) projects (NAMRU-2, 2007b).

In fiscal year 2006, there were eight AI/PI projects being conducted by NAMRU-2 in Southeast Asia. These projects were headed up by five U.S. military staff and supported by the NAMRU-2 administrative and management staff. At the time of the visit by the site team, there was a part-time DoD-GEIS coordinator in Jakarta who is scheduled to leave NAMRU-2 circa June 2007. His replacement, a veterinarian who most recently served at NAMRU-3, had been in Indonesia for approximately five months; this replacement DoD-GEIS coordinator, who will also serve part-time, is currently preparing for the transition (NAMRU-2, 2007b).

In Cambodia and Laos, NAMRU-2 paid contractors to manage the AI/PI-related projects in these satellite laboratories. With the expansion of

AI/PI activities in Cambodia, the NAMRU-2 laboratory in Phnom Penh had difficulty finding and hiring technical staff. Initial attempts to find competent technical personnel with training or experience in performing microbiologic techniques failed; as such individuals either were not available in Phnom Penh or were already working in critical positions in other laboratories (e.g., the Pasteur Institute). Recognizing the importance of not competing for the limited local technical personnel, NAMRU-2 and collaborating scientists from the Centers for Disease Control and Prevention (CDC) employed an innovative method to solve this problem. They hired a nongovernmental organization to search for competent, experienced technicians in neighboring Asian countries and imported them to live and work in Phnom Penh. The high level of competence and enthusiasm of these skilled senior technicians from Thailand and the Philippines has made its mark on the project. In order to build this capacity in Cambodia in the longer term, NAMRU-2 is also now supporting local training to increase the expertise in laboratories in the country (NAMRU-2, 2007b).

Technology and Information Management

In Jakarta, communications systems provide e-mail, Internet, fax, and telephone access. An onsite data center supplies computer systems support as well as data entry and analysis services.

The MoH of Indonesia is in the process of developing a shared database. Epidemiologic information is currently maintained at a central AI Response Center at the Indonesian CDC. Other than that, each institute involved in the diagnoses of H5N1-infected samples has maintained its own database (NAMRU-2, 2007b).

Conclusions

The site visit team was told that single-year funds received at the end of a fiscal year are very difficult to use effectively. For example, a large portion of the fiscal year 2007 salaries for scientific personnel were supposed to be funded by DoD-GEIS, but by early fiscal year 2007 no (or limited) DoD-GEIS funding had been received. If NAMRU-2 were to receive funding at the beginning of a fiscal year, so that it had an entire year to spend the funds, then officials at NAMRU-2 believe they would be able to plan and implement activities more effectively.

The team also noted the difficulty faced by NAMRU-2 scientists and leadership in trying to plan and coordinate during a time of uncertainty. This uncertainty includes the long-term status of NAMRU-2, since a new memorandum of understanding must be completed shortly with the Indonesian government in order for NAMRU-2 to continue and carry out its studies. Trying to undertake long-term planning in the face of such fundamental uncertainty is difficult.

A fundamental problem identified with respect to sustainability of the expanded pandemic influenza surveillance activities is this limited time period during which the one-year supplemental funds can be spent. Optimal expanded sustainable surveillance requires the allocation of multiple years—at least two and preferably three—of adequate support. This will allow more resources to be directed to the personnel costs of surveillance, allow local national staff to be better trained, and permit specific expanded surveillance projects to be more fully funded.

The site visit team heard varying opinions as to whether the position of a full-time DoD-GEIS coordinator is critical to the efficient administration and management of the DoD-GEIS program at NAMRU-2. Under any circumstances and however it is accomplished, significant administrative support is crucial to the management and overview of the various DoD-GEIS AI projects. Given the challenges associated with the AI/PI funds, NAMRU-2 would benefit from an additional administrator. A full-time dedicated administrative officer would be helpful to assure optimal use of DoD-GEIS funds and maximize productivity from the scientists.

SURVEILLANCE

The Influenza-Like Illness (ILI) Surveillance Project began in Indonesia in 1999. The original study, which ran from 1999 to 2004, involved six sites and was funded by DoD-GEIS. In 2004, this work was augmented with funding from the CDC, and 20 sites were subsequently established. The surveillance network was increased to 28 sites in 2005 with supplemental funding from DoD-GEIS and the U.S. Agency for International Development (NAMRU-2, 2007b).

Using the 2006 AI/PI supplemental funding, NAMRU-2's avian and pandemic influenza surveillance program was expanded to incorporate both animal and human surveillance, including surveillance of influenza viruses in migratory birds in Java; a passive surveillance network to detect influenza viruses in humans with influenza-like illness alone or with diarrhea and acute respiratory symptoms in Indonesia; and development of new human surveillance projects and diagnostic capabilities in Laos and Cambodia (NAMRU-2, 2007b). Specimens that come in for the detection of influenza virus or other respiratory pathogens are accompanied by clinical and demographic data. There is a parallel surveillance project being carried out by Litbangkes, the National Institute of Health Research and Development Laboratory, but the clinical and demographic data collected by NAMRU-2 surveillance activities provide added value. This network regularly tests over 500 human specimens a month, and has collected 697 throat swab samples and 698 cloacal swab samples from 64 species of domestic birds, resident wild birds, and migratory birds.

Human Surveillance

NAMRU-2 is implementing four protocols related to human cases of highly pathogenic influenza, including medical record review (Indonesia), prevalence of avian and human influenza viruses among diarrheal pediatric cases (Indonesia), passive hospital surveillance for acute influenza-like illness (Laos), and seroincidence in humans and seroprevalence in animals of avian influenza virus infections (Cambodia) (NAMRU-2, 2007b).

NAMRU-2's medical record review protocol is assessing severe respiratory disease among hospitalized patients across Indonesia through a systematic review of inpatient medical records. A standardized data-abstraction form, based on the common clinical manifestation of current H5N1 cases in Indonesia, was mailed to participating referral hospitals. Medical record personnel at each hospital complete questionnaires, including demographic, clinical, and laboratory data for each patient meeting the inclusion criteria (NAMRU-2, 2007b). By the study's end in 2007, NAMRU-2 plans to have collected data on medical records dated from January 2003 through December 2005. In order to identify possible H5N1 infections prior to Indonesia's first laboratory-confirmed H5N1 cases in July 2005, NAMRU-2 extended its retrospective review to roughly one year's worth of data prior to the first documented cases of H5N1 poultry infection in November 2003. NAMRU-2 will also use the data to determine if there was an increase in morbidity and mortality associated with severe respiratory disease over the same timeframe. NAMRU-2 plans to run descriptive statistics and a simple factor analysis on the data collected to identify prior H5N1 cases based on current clinical and laboratory knowledge of confirmed H5N1 cases (e.g. symptoms such as fever, pneumonia, leukopenia, lymphocytopenia, hypoalbuminia, and elevated liver enzymes). Morbidity and mortality estimates will be established based on the catchment population of the respective hospitals.

In some fatal cases of avian influenza reported in Vietnam and Thailand, diarrhea occurred without any respiratory symptoms, and laboratory testing has found that highly pathogenic avian influenza H5N1 is present in the stool of infected patients (de Jong, et al. 2005 and Wiwanitkit, 2005). Local Indonesian laboratories have also documented that diarrhea was a common symptom reported by several patients infected with highly pathogenic avian influenza H5N1 (NAMRU-2, 2007b). NAMRU-2 has developed a protocol to determine whether or not influenza A or B, especially highly pathogenic avian influenza, is shed in stool during primary influenza infections and to assess the association of viral recovery in stool versus upper respiratory specimens in the same patient. Viral RNA is extracted from stool and throat swabs collected from diarrheal pediatric patients with influenza symptoms (fever and runny or stuffy nose) who are recruited from hospitals and community health centers across Indonesia. Stool specimens and respiratory specimens are examined using multiplex nested-PCR to identify influenza A and influenza B viruses in the same reaction tube, based on two unique primer pair-sets. To date, approximately 6,000 pediatric patients have been enrolled, from which 364 matched stool-throat swabs have been collected. This study has found a high prevalence of human influenza A and B (12.1 percent) in pediatric diarrhea cases (NAMRU-2, 2007b). As this study continues NAMRU-2 researchers expect it will provide critical surveillance in detecting H5N1 in patients whose respiratory symptoms may be minimized in favor of more common gastroenteritis diagnoses.

The Laos People's Democratic Republic has had no human ILI surveillance network to identify human cases. Beginning in 2007, in conjunction with the MoH and CDC, NAMRU-2 developed a network of surveillance hospitals and clinics to screen and identify cases of H5N1 infections (NAMRU-2, 2007b). Using specific case definitions for selection purposes, ILI cases and controls are enrolled, throat and nasal swabs are obtained, and a study questionnaire is completed. At each hospital site at least 333 cases and 333 controls are required to be enrolled. Samples will be examined locally for screening purposes using rapid influenza A&B tests. At the National Center for Laboratory and Epidemiology (NCLE) in Vientiane, specimens will be screened by a multiplex system for pathogen identification. H5N1-positive specimens will be confirmed by real-time RT-PCR (reverse transcriptase polymerase chain reaction) methodology. Positive H5N1 isolates will be shipped to and characterized at the CDC and a World Health Organization (WHO) laboratory identified by the Ministry of Health (MoH) (NAMRU-2, 2007b). NAMRU-2 expects this study to yield information about influenza in Laos, to enhance Laos's capacity to identify potential pandemic influenza viruses and other highly pathogenic and virulent respiratory pathogens, and to provide the CDC with a broader net to identify highly pathogenic influenza viruses. Since MoH representatives are being trained in an extremely versatile and cost-effective diagnostic system for surveillance and outbreak investigation, NAMRU-2 also expects this project to increase the indigenous diagnostic capacity.

The widespread epizootic of avian influenza A (H5N1) that has emerged among poultry since 2003 has resulted in severe and fatal H5N1 human cases in Asia, the Middle East, the Near East, and Europe, but human deaths have not always paralleled the poultry outbreaks (WHO, 2005; FAO, 2007, WHO, 2006b). It is thought that human H5N1 influenza infections (clinical and subclinical) have occurred much more frequently than suggested. In order to increase information on H5N1 prevalence and incidence in humans and animals, NAMRU-2 will attempt to calculate the baseline seroprevalence and annual seroincidence of H1, H3, and H5 influenza virus infections in adults and animals living in a rural village in Kandal Province, Cambodia, and the seroprevalence of H5, H7, and H9 influenza virus in poultry, swine, and felines in a rural village also in Cambodia (NAMRU-2, 2007b). More than six hundred adults 18 years of age and older residing in adjacent villages in Kandal Province will be enrolled in this program. In each household, one adult will be randomly selected for enrollment. Animals—one chicken, one pig, and one cat per household—will be bled at baseline to determine seroprevalence in the same villages.

Animal Surveillance

The prevalence of the H5N1 and other avian influenza viruses in migratory birds and other animal reservoirs in Indonesia is unknown. In order to address this gap in knowledge, NAMRU-2 is supporting a multi-pronged animal influenza surveillance program in Indonesia. This program has three main objectives: to develop and conduct surveillance of avian influenza viruses in migratory and wild birds; to train Indonesian government scientists in field and laboratory techniques for collecting and testing for virus; and to use remote sensing to determine environmental correlates for transmission (NAMRU-2, 2007b).

Routine sampling of migratory and wild birds and domestic waterfowl has begun at two sites on the island of Java. Samples taken from these specimens are tested for the presence of H5N1 and other influenza A viruses. As of October 2006, NAMRU-2 had collected 695 serum samples, 697 throat swab samples, and 698 cloacal swab samples. Of these, 585 serum samples have been tested so far, and four domestic Muscovy ducks (*Cairina moschata)*, 2 plovers (*Charadrius* spp.), and samples from a purple swamphen (*Porphyrio porphyrio)* have been found to be presumptively positive for HA antibodies, that is, antibodies against influenza virus hemagglutinin. RT-PCR tests on throat and cloacal swab samples are ongoing to identify possible viruses (NAMRU-2, 2007b).

NAMRU-2 is working with the University of Iowa to coordinate training for relevant Indonesian government experts. From September 18-29, 2006, three scientists from Indonesia's Ecology and Health Status Research and Development Center, National Institute of Health Research and Development (Litbangkes) participated in didactic and laboratory training at the University of Iowa's Center for Emerging Infectious Diseases. This training focused on collection, proper handling, and testing techniques for emerging zoonotic diseases, including avian influenza.

NAMRU-2 is also collaborating with the government of Indonesia to plan for studies involving remote sensing and environmental correlates of avian influenza virus transmission. A seminar was held for the Litbangkes institute outlining the role of remote sensing in infectious disease research and control. Two of the three objectives of this study have been met. The third, involving remote sensing of environmental parameters, has been planned, and a protocol is with the Indonesian MoH awaiting approval. NAMRU-2 expects that this project will begin in fiscal year 2007.

Conclusions

The committee was impressed with the surveillance protocols implemented at NAMRU-2, particularly those involving the University of Iowa and AFRIMS, and it encourages additional collaborative activities and initiatives between DoD laboratories. In addition, the committee concluded that NAMRU-2's work with novel findings will greatly contribute to knowledge of the H5N1 influenza virus.

RECOMMENDATION 3-1. NAMRU-2 should vigorously pursue work with novel findings, e.g., influenza/diarrheal studies, which have the potential to contribute to surveillance and improve understanding of how the virus spreads.

LABORATORY

NAMRU-2 Laboratory in Indonesia

NAMRU-2 Jakarta is located in 62,000 square feet of laboratory, office, and storage spaces in three buildings within the Indonesian Ministry of Health, National Institutes of Health Research and Development (Litbangkes) compound (DoD-GEIS, 2007a). The facilities are well equipped, and the animal facility is accredited by the American Association for the Accreditation of Laboratory Animal Care. The virology laboratory capacity at NAMRU-2 includes tissue culture capabilities along with serological and molecular biological testing technologies (NAMRU-2, 2007b).

As of March 2007, there was no biosafety level-3 (BSL-3) laboratory available to NAMRU-2 or the National Institute of Health Research and Development (Litbangkes) scientists in which to attempt to culture H5 viruses under appropriate biosafety and physical containment. Consequently, there is currently no ability to do microneutralization assays for measuring anti-H5 antibody or to test the susceptibility of local H5N1 viral isolates to oseltamivir or other antiviral drugs. However, largely as a response to the H5N1 pandemic threat, two BSL-3 laboratories are expected to come online within the next two years. These include the Ejikman Institute (expected to be online by the middle of 2007) and the Litbangkes BSL-3 (which could be online in 2008). The Litbangkes leadership, NAMRU-2 scientists, U.S. embassy officials, and WHO work together closely to make arrangements for NAMRU-2 scientists to use the Litbangkes BSL-3 facility and to contribute to its maintenance.

The IOM site visit team asked whether there is an equivalent in Indonesia of a CDC BSL-3 inspection team or any established criteria to determine the suitability of the BSL-3 physical plant, its intended procedures, the credentials of proposed investigators, and the training procedures. The answer given to the site visit team was that the NAMRU-2 staff was unaware of any such controls. During a meeting with the US Embassy staff, the site visit team learned that there will be some U.S. guidance and assistance for this with respect to the Litbangkes BSL-3, but no one knew the answers to the analogous questions regarding the Ejikman BSL-3.

NAMRU-2's H5 surveillance sample testing is based mainly on RT-PCR methodology. This is done using real time RT-PCR and multiplex RT-PCR. The relative utility of these RT-PCR methodologies depends on the specific project. For example, multiplex RT-PCR is a state-of-the-art diagnostic technology that can be adapted to allow multiple important human respiratory pathogens (viral and bacterial) to be identified simultaneously. With appropriate primers encoding antigens specific for various pathogens, more than 20 individual pathogens can be identified simultaneously. As such, multiplex RT-PCR is particularly suited to broad epidemiologic studies of acute respiratory disease. Moreover, it is an extraordinarily useful tool for simultaneously determining the seasonality of an array of respiratory pathogens. However, the multiplex RT-PCR device is relatively expensive to operate. The committee was informed that the cost of processing each microtiter plate is approximately $5,262 (NAMRU-2, 2007c). Thus, the annual costs of studying seasonality by running one plate per day, five days per week, as the laboratory is currently doing, costs more than $1 million per year.

At present, presumptive H5 antibody in animal and human sera is detected at NAMRU-2 by the hemagglutination inhibition method; until a BSL-3 is available, microneutralization tests cannot be performed. The site visit team drew attention to the complexity of detecting antibodies to avian influenza viruses in mammalian sera. The NAMRU-2 laboratory also cultures H3 and H1 influenza A as well as influenza B viruses by cell-culture methods. Specimens are shared with the MoH.

The team was informed that Indonesian veterinarians working for NAMRU-2 have the capability to perform autopsies on dead birds, cats, and other animals suspected of having succumbed to H5N1 (or other) influenza viruses and that they can perform sophisticated histopathologic examinations. The technical level of competence for these pathological examinations at NAMRU-2 is high.

In briefly inspecting the laboratories, it was apparent to the IOM team that NAMRU-2 also has well-equipped and well-staffed bacteriology laboratories which can perform, as necessary, studies of secondary bacterial infections that may complicate H5 viral infections. Should pandemic disease occur, the capability to do good bacteriologic studies in patients with H5N1 disease could be extremely important since, even if a pandemic H5N1 virus were commonly to cause primary viral pneumonia (as in the 1918 pandemic), the possibility of a bacterial dimension to pulmonary infections remains.

On average, NAMRU-2 tests specimens from approximately 100 suspected H5N1 cases a month for rapid laboratory diagnosis along with other samples with suspected respiratory pathogens. Virus-positive blood or respiratory samples are shipped to the CDC for verification, genetic sequencing, sharing with the Indonesian MoH, and use in assay and vaccine development.

NAMRU-2 Laboratory in Cambodia

NAMRU-2 has a well-equipped, well-fitted physical plant for laboratory research in Phnom Penh. The NAMRU-2 building is located on the National Institute of Public Health (NIPH) campus, where several other agencies also have their administrative and technical operations. These include the Pasteur Institute of Phnom Penh, the CDC unit's offices and laboratories, and the National Institute of Public Health (NAMRU-2, 2007b).

During the IOM team's site visit, the laboratory's influenza capacity was still being established. Active training was going on and the team was able to view a training session that involved the multiplex RT-PCR machine provided to the laboratory by the DoD-GEIS supplemental funding. This laboratory is primarily responsible for providing microbiologic support to field studies. Also included in the laboratory is a DNA/RNA extractor paid for by DoD-GEIS influenza surveillance supplemental funds.

NAMRU-2 Laboratory in Laos

The site visit team did not visit Vientiane but was informed that NAMRU-2 has been working in Laos for eight years, with influenza-specific work being done in the past year and a half. This work began with regular DoD-GEIS funding, but supplemental AI monies have allowed the initiation of a new influenza surveillance study and the hiring of additional staff.

Influenza surveillance activities in Laos involve close collaboration with the NCLE in Vientiane. Specimens from patients with respiratory infections are being collected in Savannakhet and two other towns and then flown to Vientiane (NAMRU-2, 2007b).

To support these activities NAMRU-2 has put in a multiplex PCR system to detect influenza viruses and other respiratory pathogens and is looking for innovative ways to hire staff to operate the machines. The IOM site visit team learned that the multiplex PCR machine belongs to NAMRU-2 and would likely not be donated to Laos upon completion of the project. This is relevant for two reasons: First, it is usual in capacity-building to leave behind the apparatus used to perform the project and upon which people were trained; this presupposes selection of an apparatus that is technologically appropriate. Second, while there are great advantages to a multiplex PCR apparatus (as detailed above), the cost of running specimens is high and may not be sustainable by the NCLE.

Conclusions

NAMRU-2 has built upon a strong laboratory capacity in its host countries. All three facilities have benefited from improvements made with the AI/PI funds, including the addition of advanced multiplex systems in each laboratory. These systems allow the laboratories to greatly simplify certain types of epidemiologic studies, such as determining the range of pathogens seen in association with acute respiratory infections in different geographic areas. While the site visit team was impressed with the expanded capabilities this technology adds to all of the laboratories, its members did have concerns about the sustainability of this sort of advanced diagnostic system due to its high cost of operation.

RESPONSE CAPACITY

Outbreak Response

NAMRU-2 has a tradition of supporting the ministries of health in the region in investigating and responding to significant disease threats, such as severe acute respiratory syndrome (SARS) in 2003. NAMRU-2 continues to serve as a resource for Litbangkes and the other arms of the MoH as well as for the Ministry of Agriculture and Fishery in responding to epidemiologic needs, such as outbreaks of H5 in humans and birds. For example, NAMRU-2 was the first laboratory to identify H5N1 in Indonesia in July 2005, and since that time it has worked with the MoH to identify and confirm new cases. At the time of the IOM team's site visit, there had been approximately 11 clusters of cases of H5 in humans among the 78 cases of H5 in Indonesia. NAMRU-2 provided technical support to Litbangkes and other arms of the MoH in their investigation of these outbreaks. The MoH and NAMRU-2 maintained close contact with WHO in the assessment of these clusters.

NAMRU-2's role as a resource in investigation and response during outbreaks has been through an AI/PI-funded protocol focused on providing epidemiological, clinical, and laboratory support for MoH investigations of suspected or confirmed cases of H5N1 as well as suspected human or poultry outbreaks in Indonesia, Cambodia, and Laos. This funding has also allowed NAMRU-2 to deploy epidemiology teams and technicians upon request to investigation sites, to assist the ministries of health to develop appropriate investigation strategies and specimen-collection procedures, to provide laboratory diagnostic support upon request for any suspected H5N1 cases, and to train laboratory technicians in preparation for investigations.

Through these efforts, NAMRU-2 personnel were able to participate in several field investigations with the Indonesian MoH and the WHO, assisting in specimen collection and case-contact data collection for individual case and cluster investigations.

In Laos, NAMRU-2 provided rapid diagnostic kits, specimen collection supplies, and personal protective equipment to the MoH in the case-finding investigation of populations surrounding a farm with confirmed H5N1 chicken deaths. This assistance was coordinated with the CDC AI representative in Laos, and it provided critical diagnostic support to the MoH and the WHO in the identification of human and animal H5N1 cases.

Surge Capacity

Under routine conditions NAMRU-2 performs real-time RT-PCR and Luminex screening on 350 respiratory specimens per week (suspected H5N1 and other routine surveillance). Additionally, the laboratory in Cambodia currently screens 10 respiratory specimens per week using real-time RT-PCR, although since this surveillance project was started just in December 2006, the number of specimens is expected to increase (NAMRU-2, 2007a). The laboratory in Laos is not yet operational but is expected to be shortly. The total number of specimens processed at the three NAMRU-2 facilities is approximately 360 per week (see Table 3-1).

If the algorithm was altered to first test influenza A and then, if positive, to test H5, NAMRU-2 facilities would be able to test 4,900 specimens per week. The Jakarta laboratory would be able to increase specimen testing to 3,400 specimens per week (2,000 using real-time RT-PCR and an additional 1,400 using the Luminex technology); the Phnom Penh laboratory would be able to test 1,000 specimens per week (500 using real-time RT-PCR and an additional 500 using the Luminex technology); and the Laos laboratory, if requested to do testing for a suspected outbreak, could test 500 specimens per week (NAMRU-2, 2007a).

If the algorithm was altered further to target only the gene required to

TABLE 3-1 Summary of Surge Capability at NAMRU-2

Condition	Indonesia (# specimens/week)		Cambodia (# specimens/week)		Laos (# specimens/week)		Total (# specimens/ week)
	rt RT-PCR	Luminex	rt RT-PCR	Luminex	rt RT-PCR	Luminex	
Routine operation	AI Suspect: 75 ILI: 250	Normal operations 25	AI: 0 ILI: 10		Pending protocol approval	Pending protocol approval	360
Altered algorithm influenza A and H5 first	2,000	1,400	500	500	To be implemented this FY	500	4,900
Target only specific gene	3,000	1,400	700	500	To be implemented this FY	500	11,000
24-hours-a-day, seven-days-a-week operations	5,000	8,000	1,200	2,500	To be implemented this FY	2,500	19,200

NOTE: Multiplex bead-based assay for simultaneous screening against 19 viral pathogens, including FLU A matrix and H1, H3, and H5.
SOURCE: NAMRU-2, 2007a.

identify the strain of interest, then NAMRU-2 facilities could process up to 11,000 specimens a week. In Jakarta, 4,400 specimens could be tested a week (3,000 using real-time RT-PCR and an additional 1,400 using the Luminex technology); the Phnom Penh laboratory would be able to test 1,200 specimens per week (700 using real-time RT-PCR and an additional 500 using the Luminex technology); and the Laos laboratory, if requested to do testing for a suspected outbreak, could test 500 specimens per week. The limiting factor here would be sustainability of reagents and supplies on hand.

If NAMRU-2 transitioned to a 24-hours-a-day, 7–days-a-week operation, NAMRU-2 facilities could process up to 19,200 specimens a week. In Jakarta, 13,000 specimens could be tested a week (5,000 using real-time RT-PCR and an additional 8,000 using the Luminex technology); the Phnom Penh laboratory would be able to test 3,700 specimens per week (1,200 using real-time RT-PCR and an additional 2,500 using the Luminex technology); and the Laos laboratory, if requested to do testing for a suspected outbreak, could test 2,500 specimens per week (NAMRU-2, 2007a). Implementation of surge-capacity operations in Cambodia and Laos will be limited by personnel and resources.

NAMRU-2 does not stockpile reagents, as would be necessary to handle these sample loads for prolonged periods. Thus reagents would have to be acquired on an emergency basis to carry out work at this volume. This would present a logistics problem, as replenishment of supplies can normally take from 3 to 6 months during routine operations.

In addition, intrinsic limitations on personnel resources in Cambodia and Laos will limit the quantity of specimens tested. Technicians are cross-trained to use both real-time PCR and multiplex systems, but they cannot do both at the same time.

Conclusions

Outbreak response activities in Indonesia have demonstrated to the MoH as well as to the Ministry of Agriculture and Fishery the benefits that NAMRU-2 provides to the country and the region. The IOM team pondered what the role of NAMRU-2 and DoD-GEIS would have in responding to the onset of a major epidemic of a new influenza virus. The history of the relationship between the government of Indonesia and NAMRU-2 has been that in the time of health or civil crises—for example, the 2004 tsunami or the Yogyakarta earthquake—the Government has called upon the U.S. Navy to provide assistance, and NAMRU-2 has responded rapidly and effectively. The effectiveness of response to a future pandemic will depend in large part on how soon such a pandemic might arrive, as Litbangkes and NAMRU-2 need a certain amount of time to have their diagnostic technologies well in place to handle such an outbreak. NAMRU-2 would have much to offer in its ability to cope with a surge situation, especially in the early stages of a pandemic.

There do not appear to be too many other ways that NAMRU-2 can assist the health systems to respond to an influenza pandemic. There are few clinicians on the NAMRU-2 staff and little equipment that would be relevant. Its support would be provided mainly through technical assistance, and clinical training. More importantly, NAMRU-2 could provide diagnostic input to let the ministry know that the epidemic to which their health systems must respond is in fact pandemic influenza. The committee would see this as valuable input from NAMRU-2 in the event that this does occur, and deeper links with the ministry could be forged as part of a significant contribution to influenza pandemic preparedness.

CAPACITY BUILDING

NAMRU-2 has purchased equipment and supplies for its laboratory and collaborating laboratories in Southeast Asia in order to support ongoing surveillance activities, increase surge capacity, augment molecular diagnostic capability, and provide the means to rapidly test multiple specimens for influenza A H5N1 and to rapidly sequence samples from patients with confirmed H5N1 infection.

An automated nucleic acid extractor was purchased for the NAMRU-2 laboratory in Indonesia to assist in sample processing. Additional thermocyclers have allowed for the simultaneous amplification of multiple targets for hundreds of samples at the same time. An ABI 3300 gene sequencer has been added to the new molecular virology laboratory, and, in addition, funds provided for this project have supported the purchase of reagents and the hiring of two technicians to oversee activities.

NAMRU-2 has provided the laboratory in Phnom Penh, Cambodia, with significant support in the form of equipment, supplies, and personnel with which to conduct avian influenza projects in the country. Examples include an automated nucleic acid extractor to assist in sample processing and a real-time RT-PCR machine for the analysis of multiple targets and samples; a multiplex instrument, installed and commissioned in the NIPH/NAMRU-2 laboratory in Phnom Penh; temperature-sensitive reagents to run about 1,000 samples; the hiring of a contract laboratory technician, trained by NAMRU-2 staff, as well as equipment distributor staff; and the purchase of proficiency panels in collaboration with the Naval Health Research Center (NHRC), which will be used to establish a quarterly quality assurance/quality control (QA/QC) program for the laboratory.

In Vientiane, Laos, NAMRU-2 has provided the same as it has in Phnom Penh, with the exception of the nucleic acid extractor.

In addition, NAMRU-2 is funding the development of a Singapore location in order to attract potential research partners based in Singapore, establish a base for diagnostic and training operations, enhance logistical capabilities and operational agility for surveillance activities in Cambodia, Laos, and Indonesia, and serve as a strategic training unit, capable of providing training to NAMRU-2 regional partners. As part of the establishment of this platform, NAMRU-2 expects to install a multiplex system at the Defense Science Organization (DSO) National Laboratories at Kent Ridge in Singapore. Furthermore, NAMRU-2 sponsored a symposium at DSO National Laboratories, which brought together delegates from the Indonesia, Laos, Cambodia, and Singapore ministries of health to discuss disease surveillance and evaluation of detection platforms. This project is ongoing.

Conclusions

NAMRU-2 has invested in building the capacity of all three of their partner facilities. The IOM site visit team learned that the large items of equipment purchased with supplemental influenza surveillance monies, including the multiplex PCR apparatus installed in Cambodia and Laos, represent Department of the Navy equipment that would not be left behind should the influenza surveillance budget be severely curtailed. IOM site visitors were informed that this lack of transfer of ownership of the equipment to host country institutions was clearly explained to host country collaborators. Moreover, even if the expensive pieces of equipment, such as the multiplex system, were transferred to the host country institutions, the cost of operation of these machines is almost certainly too prohibitive to be sustained by the local authorities. For example, the IOM committee was informed that one 96-well plate tested in the multiplex system at NAMRU-2 in Jakarta costs $5,262 to process (NAMRU-2, 2007c).

Importantly, with respect to both running the current projects and capacity building, these experienced senior technical staff are training a cadre of Khmer technicians. The site visit team watched a training session in which Khmer trainees were being taught to operate a multiplex apparatus. During the site visit to Phnom Penh, the IOM team learned that within the local technical school some Cambodian students are trained each year as laboratory technicians. However, the training is in French, and these graduates, who speak only Khmer and French, would have difficulty communicating in a laboratory where the technical supervisors and investigators speak English but not Khmer or French. For some projects this would not be a major problem, but because of the diagnostic ramifications of H5 surveillance there has been reluctance to hire non-English speaking technical staff.

COLLABORATION AND COORDINATION

Collaborative relationships between organizations and agencies with public health interests in Indonesia (including agencies of the Indonesian government, the U.S. government, and international organizations) are quite complex. Within Indonesia, NAMRU-2 has been working closely with Litbangkes and the Ministry of Agriculture and Fishery with respect to influenza surveillance. While relationships on a technical level are collaborative, there have been a couple of issues related to the flow of results and samples which, at the time of the IOM visit, had recently affected both NAMRU-2's relationship with the government and the laboratory's ability to function effectively. While these issues appear to have been resolved, they highlight the importance of transparency and of collaboration with host governments.

One of these issues was related to the flow of samples and results to reference laboratories outside of Indonesia. Respiratory specimens collected by NAMRU-2 were conventionally split into several aliquots, one of which was sent to Litbangkes for testing there. In addition, specimens that tested positive for H5 in the NAMRU-2 laboratory were sent to the CDC in Atlanta, a WHO international reference center, for confirmation and sequence analysis. Prior to March 2006, the CDC standard operating procedure was to send confirmation and sequence information only to the laboratory that provided the specimen and not routinely to the ministry of health of the host country where the submitting laboratory resided. Because NAMRU-2 was inadvertently receiving information before the Indonesia MoH, this created a delicate situation. The issue was resolved when CDC agreed to report results simultaneously to NAMRU-2 and to Litbangkes.

The other issue related to another CDC standard operating procedure, which was to make viral isolates available upon request to manufacturers of influenza vaccines for humans and to make the sequences publicly available to everyone in Genbank. This was in accordance with the rules of the WHO International Influenza Reference Laboratories, but the Indonesian government was unhappy with the way its viruses and sequences were being handled, and it argued that a lack of respect was being shown for the needs of Indonesia as a sovereign government. This issue became complicated when CSL (the Australian producer of influenza vaccines) prepared a candidate H5N1 vaccine, based on an Indonesian isolate sequence obtained from GenBank, by using reverse genetics to create a vaccine seed virus strain expressing the hemagglutinin antigen of this recent Indonesian virus that could be grown to high titer in eggs. When CSL announced the development of the vaccine and this was brought to the attention of Indonesia's MoH, the information was misinterpreted, and it was concluded that somehow CSL had physically obtained Indonesian H5 isolates without the knowledge of the Indonesian government.

These vaccine-related points of contention were aggravated by several other instances, described to the team by senior MoH officials, in which Indonesian isolate sequence data were presented at international conferences without Indonesian scientists or the Indonesian government being informed. Collectively, these incidents led the MoH of Indonesia to declare that the country would no longer send H5 isolates to WHO reference labs, nor would it share sequence data. This created an international crisis with respect to surveillance activities for H5 in Indonesia (currently the site of most reported human cases globally), and it also seriously impaired surveillance activities at NAMRU-2. The site visit team was in Indonesia in the midst of this very complicated, difficult situation with its implications for global surveillance for H5.

An important clarification was provided to the site visit team when it visited with the WHO country representative in Jakarta. He indicated that at the highest levels of WHO there was involvement and discussions with the Minister of Health of Indonesia and with her associates over the issues of sending virus isolates to a WHO influenza reference laboratory and sharing strains and sequence data. The site visit team was told that in early March the Director General of WHO sent a letter to the Minister of Health of Indonesia clearly stating WHO's position that the specimens of Indonesian origin would be used only for risk assessment and not vaccine manufacture (i.e., for non-commercial purposes) and strongly urging the country to once again send strains to a WHO international influenza reference laboratory. The IOM team was informed that a letter of reply from the Indonesian government to WHO had been sent but WHO had not yet seen it. However, it was implied that the basic agreement was in place to allow resumption of the export of H5 isolates to WHO influenza reference laboratories. A high-level technical conference was being convened on an urgent basis for the week of March 27, and it was expected that this conference would accomplish useful technical exchange.

In response to the Indonesian government's concerns, WHO held a two-day meeting in March 2007. According to WHO, the meeting discussions focused on striking a balance between the need to continue the sharing of influenza viruses for risk assessment and for vaccine development and the need to ensure that developing countries benefit from sharing. The WHO collaborating centers will continue to perform risk assessment on H5N1 virus samples and to transform virus into seed virus suitable for vaccine production. Following discussion with representatives of the Indonesian MoH, these processes will be documented in a revised terms of reference for the WHO laboratories. Following this meeting, the MoH of Indonesia announced that the country would immediately resume the sharing of H5N1 avian influenza virus samples. In addition, the World Health Assembly in May of 2007 reiterated the importance of sharing virus samples as well as ensuring that developing countries are involved in and benefit from the global surveillance network (WHA, 2007).

As demonstrated by the handling of the recent problem with the Indonesian government, NAMRU-2 works closely with WHO. During the IOM team's visit, its members met with officials from the WHO, who confirmed that NAMRU-2 is well coordinated with and closely linked with WHO activities.

As mentioned previously, specimens positive for H5N1 and other influenza viruses are shipped immediately to the CDC for confirmation and genetic analysis, if applicable. In collaboration with the National Aeronautics and Space Administration, data from animal surveillance will be coordinated with satellite data to determine environmental correlates for transmission of AI.

NAMRU-2 creates weekly updates on H5N1 in Indonesia, which are made available to the DoD-GEIS Headquarters and the U.S. embassy in Jakarta. In the last two years, this program has received funding from DoD-GEIS, CDC, and the U.S Agency for International Development.

Sources at the U.S. embassy were highly complimentary of the NAMRU-2 influenza surveillance system and overall technical capabilities, and they specifically mentioned how embassy officials have repeatedly received phone calls and cables from congressional offices asking specific questions about the H5 situation in Indonesia. The NAMRU-2 staff have been invaluable in providing up-to-date, objective responses on a round-the-clock basis. Therefore the NAMRU-2 surveillance system and the NAMRU-2 technical personnel have been an extremely useful resource to the U.S. embassy.

Finally, in collaboration with the Armed Forces Research Institute of Medical Sciences (AFRIMS), NAMRU-2 scientists are involved in influenza surveillance activities in Thailand. In undertaking this collaboration, the scientists provided training in influenza A H5N1 diagnostic assays to the AFRIMS laboratory personnel in Bangkok to establish and standardize these tests.

Conclusions

GEIS is integrated with current, ongoing activities within Indonesia's public health infrastructure. Within-country relationships are largely person based and proximity driven, and strong partnerships have resulted over the years. NAMRU-2 DoD-GEIS staff seemed very well known and respected by the national health authorities. The interaction between NAMRU-2 and the Litbangkes staff is strong. The Ministry of Health, primarily Litbangkes, approves all projects funded by GEIS. DoD-GEIS activities are transparent to the Indonesian Ministry of Health, and most projects are jointly conducted.

NAMRU-2 also works closely with relevant government agencies on influenza surveillance activities in Cambodia and Laos. The site visit team felt that NAMRU-2 was working well in all of its locations, even in the face of serious challenges to coordination. In spite of the period of uncertainty with respect to a new long-term memorandum of understanding with the government of Indonesia, the committee supported NAMRU-2's continued support and expansion of influenza surveillance activities in neighboring countries.

NAMRU-2's ongoing collaboration with AFRIMS allows for improved utilization of AI/PI resources as well as redundant coverage for each of the laboratories in the event of a crisis (political, geologic, etc.) that might close one and not the other during a pandemic.

RECOMMENDATION 3-2. NAMRU-2 should continue to strengthen its relationship with AFRIMS and to coordinate DoD-GEIS influenza activities in the region.

REFERENCES

DoD-GEIS (Department of Defense Global Emerging Infections System). 2007a. *U.S. Naval Medical Research Unit No. 2*. http://www.geis.fhp.osd.mil/GEIS/Training/namru-2asp.asp (accessed June 12, 2007)

DoD-GEIS. 2007b. *Department of Defense influenza surveillance sites worldwide, 2007* (unpublished).

de Jong, M. D., Cam, B. V., Qui, P. T., Hien, V. M., Thanh, T. T., Hue, N. B., Beld, M., Phuong, L. T., Khanh, T. H., Chau, N. V. V., Hien, T. T., Ha, D. Q., Farrar, J. 2005. Fatal avian influenza A (H5N1) in a child presenting with diarrhea followed by coma. *New England Journal of Medicine* 352:686-691.

FAO (Food and Agricultural Organization of the United Nations). 2007. *Combining poultry vaccination with other disease control measures to combat H5N1*. http://www.fao.org/newsroom/en/news/2007/1000527/index.html (accessed June 12, 2007).

Naipospos, T.S.P. 2007. *The Indonesian response plan to avian influenza*. PowerPoint presented at Seasonal and Pandemic Influenza Meeting, February 1. Arlington, VA.

NAMRU-2 (Naval Medical Research Unit No. 2). 2007a. *Sample surge capacity plan* (unpublished).

NAMRU-2. 2007b. *Fiscal year 2006 AI/PI GEIS project information* (unpublished).

NAMRU-2. 2007c. *Estimated Cost of Assays* (unpublished).

WHA (World Health Assembly). 2007. *Pandemic influenza preparedness: Sharing of influenza viruses and access to vaccines and other benefits (WHA60.28)*. World Health Organization Geneva, Switzerland.

WHO (World Health Organization). 2005. *Avian influenza frequently asked questions*. http://www.who.int/csr/disease/avian_influenza/avian_faqs/en/index.html (accessed June 12, 2007).

WHO. 2006a. *Avian influenza—situation in Indonesia—update 14*. http://www.who.int/csr/don/2006_05_23/en/index.html (accessed June 12, 2007).

WHO. 2006b. *Influenza research at the human and animal interface. Report of a WHO working group*. Geneva, Switzerland 21–22 September 2006. http://www.who.int/csr/resources/publications/influenza/WHO_CDS_EPR_GIP_2006_3C.pdf (accessed July 30, 2007).

WHO. 2007a. *H5N1 avian influenza: Timeline of major events*. http://www.who.int/csr/disease/avian_influenza/Timeline_2007_03_20.pdf (accessed September 5, 2007).

WHO. 2007b. *Avian influenza outbreaks in South-East Asia*. http://www.searo.who.int/EN/section10/section1027.htm (accessed June 12, 2007).

Wiwanitkit, V. 2005. Diarrhoea as a presentation of bird flu infection: A summary on its correlation to outcome in Thai cases. *Gut* 54: 1506-1506.

LIST OF CONTACTS

DoD-GEIS NAMRU-2 Assessment: Indonesia

Patrick Blaire, Viral Disease Program, Naval Medical Research Unit No. 2, Jakarta, Indonesia
Timothy Burgess, Naval Medical Research Unit No. 2, Jakarta, Indonesia
Jonathan Glass, Naval Medical Research Unit No. 2, Jakarta, Indonesia
Herman Kosasih, Naval Medical Research Unit No. 2, Jakarta, Indonesia
Craig Stoops, Naval Medical Research Unit No. 2, Jakarta, Indonesia
Agustinalka Susanti, Luminex System, Naval Medical Research Unit No. 2, Jakarta, Indonesia
Steven Tobias, Naval Medical Research Unit No. 2, Jakarta, Indonesia
William A. Heidt, Economic Section, Embassy of the United States, Jakarta, Indonesia
Colette Marcellin, Environment, Science, Technology, and Health, Embassy of the United States, Jakarta, Indonesia
Lisa Kramer, Office of Health Population and Nutrition, United States Agency for International Development, Jakarta, Indonesia
Sardikin Giriputro, Sulianty Saroso Infectious Disease Hospital, Republic of Indonesia Ministry of Health, Jakarta, Indonesia
Triono Soendoro, Republic of Indonesia Ministry of Health, National Institute of Health Research and Development, Jakarta, Indonesia
Endang R. Sedyaningsih Mamahit, Center for Biomedical and Pharmaceutical Research and Development, National Institute of Health Research and Development, Jakarta, Indonesia
Georg Peterson, World Health Organization, Jakarta, Indonesia
Kumara Rai, World Health Organization, Jakarta, Indonesia
Helen Louise Taylor, World Health Organization, Jakarta, Indonesia

DoD-GEIS NAMRU-2 Assessment: Cambodia

Shannon Putnam, Director, Bacterial Diseases Program, Naval Medical Research Unit No. 2, Phnom Penh, Cambodia
Thomas Wierzba, Phnom Penh Laboratory, Naval Medical Research Unit No. 2, Phnom Penh, Cambodia
Bill Brady, Avian Influenza Country Coordination, National Institute of Public Health, Phnom Penh, Cambodia
Ung Sam Un, National Institute of Public Health, Phnom Penh, Cambodia

SCHEDULE OF EVENTS
DoD-GEIS NAMRU-2 Assessment

Jakarta, Indonesia and Phnom Penh, Cambodia
Participants: Dr. Myron M. Levine
Dr. Kennedy Shortridge
Kimberly Weingarten
March 5, 2007–March 10, 2007

Monday, March 5, 2007

0830-0900	**In-brief with command and scientific director**
0900-0930	**Overview of GEIS/NAMRU-2 programs** Dr. Jonathan Glass Dr. Steven Tobias
0930-1200	**Meeting with individual projects' primary investigators for 45 minutes each, including tour** Dr. Jonathan Glass and Dr. Steven Tobias, Emerging Diseases Ika Susanti, Immunology Dr. Craig Stoops and Dr. Steven Tobias, Entomology and Zoonotic Diseases
1200-1300	Lunch
1300-1500	**Meeting with individual projects' primary investigators for 45 minutes each, including tour** Dr. Patrick Blair and Dr. Timothy Burgess, Virology
1515-	**Meeting** Dr. Endang R. Sedyaningsih Mamahit, National Institutes of Health Research and Development
1900-	Dinner

Tuesday, March 6, 2007

0900-1100	**Meeting** Dr. Kumara Rai, World Health Organization Dr. George Peterson, World Health Organization
1100-1230	**Meeting** Colette Marcellin, U.S. Embassy Avian Influenza Working Group
1230-1400	Lunch
1400-	**Rumah Sakit Pneyakit Infeksi Sulianti Saroso Hospital for Influenza site visit**

Wednesday, March 7, 2007

0930-1715	Travel to Phnom Penh, Cambodia
1900-	Dinner

Thursday, March 8, 2007

0800-0845	**Meeting** Dr. Shannon Putman, Bacteriology
0845-0915	Travel to NAMRU-2 laboratory at the National Institutes of Public Health
0915-1000	**In-brief** Dr. Thomas Weirzba, Laboratory Director
1000-1100	**Tour of facility**
1100-1200	**Meeting** Dr. Bill Brady, Coordinator of Avian and Pandemic Influenza
1200-1300	Lunch
1300-1400	**Site visit to Chey Chummas Referral Hospital (Kandal Province)**
1430-1600	**Visited family farm south of Phnom Penh**
1900-	Dinner

Friday, March 9, 2007

0830-1600	Fly to Bangkok, Thailand

Saturday, March 10, 2007

1000-1640	Departure

4

Armed Forces Research Institute of Medical Sciences Thailand Avian and Pandemic Influenza Activities

The Armed Forces Research Institute of Medical Sciences (AFRIMS) in Bangkok, Thailand was established in 1958 through an agreement between the governments of the United States and Thailand. The original laboratory was created as the Cholera Research Laboratory of the Southeast Asia Treaty Organization (SEATO). The laboratory was expanded in 1961 to include research on other tropical diseases and was renamed the SEATO Medical Research Laboratory. SEATO was dissolved in 1977, and the U.S. component of AFRIMS was reorganized as a medical research laboratory run jointly by the Royal Thai Army and the U.S. Army under the overall command of a Royal Thai Army officer of flag rank. Historically, AFRIMS has been closely linked with a Royal Thai Army laboratory and also collaborates with various other national institutions, including the Thai Ministry of Health (Department of Medical Sciences, National Institute of Health, Department of Communicable Disease Control, and the Office of the Permanent Secretary and its Field Epidemiology Training Program) and the Ministry of Agriculture (Department of Livestock Development).

For many years, AFRIMS was devoted exclusively to applied research in support of its medical mission. It has successfully developed research programs with a special emphasis on the development of diagnostic tests and therapeutic products for malaria and other tropical febrile illnesses. AFRIMS research programs in infectious diseases, including diarrheal disease, malaria vaccine and drug research, viral diseases (specifically, dengue fever and hepatitis), entomology and disease vector research, and retrovirology (including human immunodeficiency virus infection and AIDS), existed long before the introduction of the Department of Defense Global Emerging Infections Surveillance and Response System (DoD-GEIS). In some ways DoD-GEIS represented a departure for AFRIMS, although in other ways DoD-GEIS is a natural extension of the field research that has been AFRIMS's mainstay. For example, the DoD-GEIS malaria pillar complements ongoing surveillance for antimalarial drug resistance, whereas surveillance for acute febrile illness is a somewhat new area of involvement.

On July 4, 2005, AFRIMS was also designated a World Health Organization (WHO) Collaborating Center for Diagnostic Reference, Training, and Investigation of Emerging Infectious Diseases. The projects undertaken by AFRIMS using the fiscal year 2006 AI/PI supplemental funding included increasing the laboratory infrastructure and capabilities of AFRIMS laboratories in Bangkok, Thailand, as well as performing regional influenza surveillance, particularly for highly pathogenic avian influenza (see Figure 4-1).

A site visit team of the Institute of Medicine (IOM) Committee for the Assessment of DoD-GEIS Influenza Surveillance and Response Programs visited AFRIMS from March 12-17, 2007.[1] The IOM site visit team spent two days in Bangkok and two and a half days in Kathmandu, Nepal, visiting the laboratories and reviewing surveillance projects supported by the DoD-GEIS supplemental funding. A list of the people with whom the site visit team met and the itinerary that was followed can be found at the end of this chapter.

INFLUENZA IN THAILAND

In January 2004, Thailand issued its first report of highly pathogenic avian influenza virus of the H5N1 subtype in poultry and humans (WHO, 2007a). Since that time Thailand has had a total of 25 human cases of avian influenza, 17 of which were fatal, but it has reported no human infections since September 2006 (although it did confirm H5N1 in poultry during routine intensive surveillance in January 2007) (WHO 2007a, WHO 2007b). In addition to its human and poultry infections, Thailand has also had a number of domestic cats, captive tigers, and leopards die of the H5N1 virus (Tiensin et al., 2005).

Other novel findings related to avian influenza in Thailand have been documented, dating back to July 2004, when a report described an atypical human H5N1 infection that lacked the usual respiratory symptoms

[1]Prior to the committee's AFRIMS visit, the laboratory staff provided the committee with detailed background information on AFRIMS and the pandemic/avian influenza activities it was supporting. These materials are available from the IOM in the Public Access File.

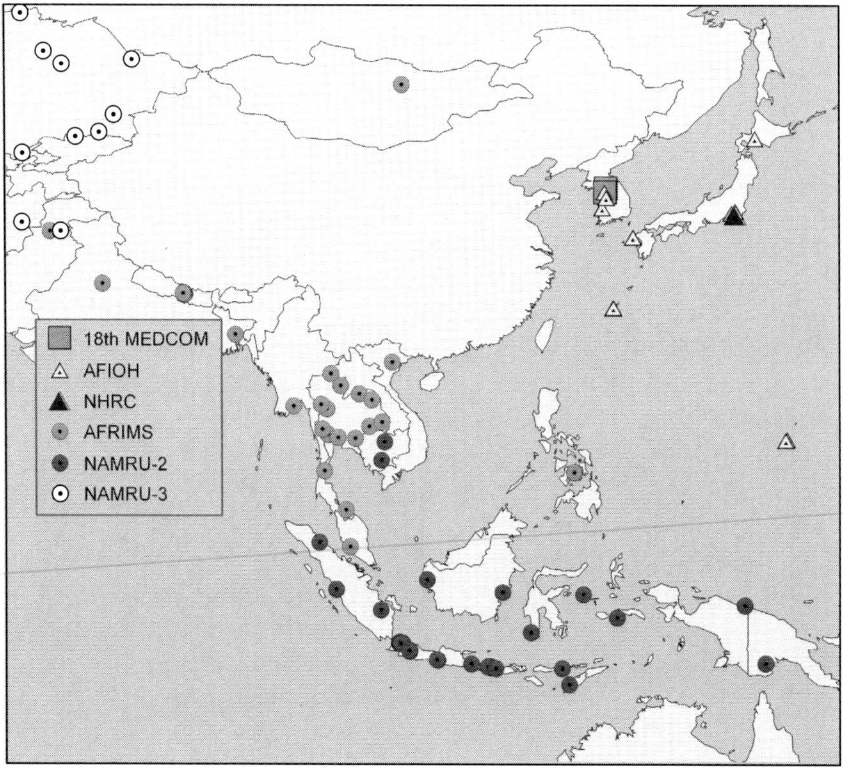

FIGURE 4-1 DoD's regional presence in influenza surveillance (South East Asia), 2007.
SOURCE: DoD-GEIS, 2007b.

and therefore indicated that the clinical spectrum of disease was perhaps broader than originally thought (Apisarnthanarak, et al. 2004). Six months later, in January 2005, the first account of a probable secondary human transmission of avian influenza resulting in severe disease was published after a young girl in Thailand was believed to have fatally infected her mother with H5N1 (WHO, 2004).

In addition to Thailand, eight countries in South and Southeast Asia have reported highly pathogenic avian influenza among poultry: Bangladesh, Cambodia, India, Indonesia, Laos, Malaysia, Myanmar, and Vietnam. Bangladesh and Myanmar both reported their first outbreaks of highly pathogenic H5N1 in poultry in early 2007. Indonesia, on the other hand, reported its first human case of H5N1 avian influenza in July 2005 and has had the highest number of AI cases worldwide (WHO 2007a, WHO 2007c).

MANAGEMENT AND PLANNING

AFRIMS's overall strategy integrates DoD-GEIS activities into traditional research streams in order to leverage AFRIMS's resources and expertise that are already in place so as to reduce program overhead costs and to complement the activities of the Thai government. This integration results in more than 80 percent of DoD-GEIS funds being allocated to program implementation rather than overhead costs. In addition, this integration complements and reflects the activities of the Thai government.

Staffing

AFRIMS employs more than 400 personnel, including 25 Americans, twelve of whom are scientists. The DoD-GEIS program is coordinated by a full-time military public health/preventive medicine officer as well as a full-time influenza program manager (Henry Jackson Foundation contract). Together they oversee the work of DoD-GEIS staff (24 in Thailand and 23 in Nepal). In addition to laboratory expertise, staff members have expertise in training (both in Bangkok and the regional countries), public relations, data processing, database design, and secretarial support. Overall the IOM team found DoD-GEIS staff members to be capable, enthusiastic about their work, and eager to develop their influenza surveillance program.

Conclusions

While AFRIMS made appropriate use of the supplemental funding, the site visit team concluded that a minimum of two years of funding for supplemental influenza surveillance is desirable, and a five-year funding package would be ideal. Ideally, a novel, modest, and stable funding stream would be created to allow for proper planning and program implementation as well as for surge capacity in the face of an unexpected outbreak situation. This would require a different approach to the proposal process structure, an approach that would ideally be applied to all OCONUS (outside of the Continental U.S.) and CONUS (Continental U.S.) laboratories.

SURVEILLANCE

AFRIMS has been involved in specimen collection as part of the DoD Influenza Surveillance Program since 1996 (AFRIMS, 2007a). Approximately one-third of the samples submitted have been positive for at least one respiratory virus in the testing panel (adenovirus, herpes simplex virus, enterovirus, influenza A and B, and parainfluenza 1, 2, and 3). Approximately 45 percent of the isolates were influenza B and 46 percent influenza A. The hemagglutinin of one of the H3 isolates submitted to the Air Force Institute for Operational Health (AFIOH) from the field site in Sangklaburi early in 2007 had an unusual amino acid change at position 142, from a glycine to arginine; this change has been noted only twice in the past two years, one in a fatal case (AFIOH, 2004).

In fiscal year 2006, AFRIMS's department of virology was able to expand its surveillance network to a total of 13 sites in five countries. It processed 490 samples (AFRIMS, 2006). These included specimens received from two influenza outbreaks in Nepal, confirmatory testing for the WHO influenza surveillance program in Nepal, and results from the U.S. embassy surveillance project.

AFRIMS's situation in Thailand has required a complementary approach as the country has its own influenza virus surveillance program and its response to the introduction of AI has been substantial. The Thai laboratory, which is affiliated with the Ministry of Public Health (MoPH), has sophisticated methodology to serve the country and is backed up at 14 remote sites across the country, all of which are also equipped with rapid testing technologies. Its internet-based reporting system will eventually merge with another AFRIMS-supported project, linking MoPH and the Ministry of Agriculture and Cooperatives to allow sharing of data on zoonotic illnesses between ministries at the provincial and national levels. Therefore, AFRIMS's capacity for AI must be directed at less well resourced countries in the region and at supplying services that are complementary to those available in Thailand.

Sentinel surveillance projects are of two types, those directed toward detection of disease in personnel of 14 regional U.S. embassies and those aimed at detecting disease in populations in Southeast Asia. In the case of the former, specimen transport has been expensive and burdensome, with small numbers tested. However, the program should have a stabilizing function should PI threaten employees.

Within Thailand, AFRIMS is expanding influenza surveillance programs through its relationship with the Royal Thai Army (AFRIMS, 2007a). In these locations, previously unaddressed by the MoPH, AFRIMS's DoD-GEIS funding supports the capacities of ten military and two civilian hospitals to detect and report influenza primarily among refugee populations and non-Thai citizens along the western border with Myanmar. This work supplements the surveillance system of the MoPH in Thailand.

In the Philippines the purpose of the AFRIMS work is to develop an active influenza surveillance program in the Cebu Province (AFRIMS, 2007a). The Philippines is beginning to incorporate this network into the national surveillance program. As in Nepal and Thailand, the protocol for influenza-like illnesses (ILI) that is employed here involves local rapid testing and followup testing by PCR (polymerase chain reaction) in Bangkok, with confirmatory testing at AFIOH in San Antonio, Texas, and selected isolates sent to the WHO Influenza Reference Laboratory at CDC in Atlanta.

Conclusions

The Committee concluded that AFRIMS's influenza surveillance protocol activities and initiatives expanded with supplemental funding represented a significant contribution to the influenza surveillance network in the region. In addition, the committee concluded that AFRIMS would greatly extend its contribution to knowledge of the H5N1 influenza virus with additional protocols focused on seasonal influenza and novel findings.

RECOMMENDATION 4-1. AFRIMS should establish more intensified surveillance for seasonal and novel strains of influenza at sites in temperate and tropical/subtropical parts of Nepal, in locales with commercial poultry production units, and at migratory bird resting sites.

LABORATORY

In Bangkok, AFRIMS occupies a total of six separate buildings at two sites approximately one kilometer apart (DoD-GEIS, 2007a). Relevant to the DOD-GEIS work, these buildings house laboratory space as well as a veterinary animal wing and a veterinary medicine building. AFRIMS is in the process of constructing a Biosafety Level 3 (BSL-3) laboratory suite. A significant deficit in the region is the availability of sufficient biosafety capacity. Funding was made available in fiscal year 2006 for AI/PI, and AFRIMS took advantage of this to build infrastructure in the form of this BSL-3 laboratory.

Real-time PCR using the RotoGene system has been established at the AFRIMS respiratory pathogen section and at the Department of Veterinary Medicine BSL-3 laboratory. AFIOH and the CDC have provided probes, primers, and training. Current capabilities include universal A and B, H1, H3, and H5 detection. Mass-tag PCR assays have also been established at AFRIMS for the identification of a range of respiratory pathogens. Study personnel and other interested personnel (both the Royal Thai Army and U.S. Army Materiel Command) will receive training on the standard operating procedures for these PCR assays.

AFRIMS is playing an important role outside of Thailand as well, primarily through the Walter Reed/AFRIMS Research Unit Nepal (WARUN). WARUN was formally established in August 1995 and currently provides influenza diagnostic support and training to various entities in Nepal, such as the National Public Health Laboratory (NPHL), the Epidemiology and Disease Control Division (EDCD), and WHO Nepal.

The WARUN laboratory has capacity for bacteriologic culture and will be fully functional in performing influenza virus PCR assays for AI/PI by June 2007. In this effort a study will be conducted with the MoPH and several clinical sites looking at ILI. Specimens will be tested at the site of collection using rapid tests, and companion specimens will be transported to WARUN for PCR testing. The results will be confirmed at the AFRIMS laboratory in Bangkok and further characterized at AFIOH in San Antonio, Texas.

Conclusions

AFRIMS has proposed a plan to rapidly accelerate its protocol for releasing PCR results in Nepal, the Philippines, and Thailand and for releasing cultures in Bangkok by January 1, 2008. Inherent in this is the need for AFRIMS to be entirely self-sufficient in its isolation and identification systems as soon as possible so that rapid and accurate results are immediately available for decision makers. AFRIMS's proposed expansion of laboratory capacity and increased autonomy would also increase its status in Thailand, a country with significant influenza resources but lacking sufficient biosafety capacity. As the facilities move toward self-sufficiency it would be beneficial to have a safety officer, in lieu of a staff member, who is responsible for laboratory containment facilities, as well as an individual devoted to the oversight of quality assurance.

RECOMMENDATION 4-2. AFRIMS should continue to work toward self-sufficiency in its isolation and identification systems in order to release PCR results more quickly to its national partners while taking appropriate steps to ensure laboratory containment and quality assurance.

RESPONSE CAPACITY

Under routine conditions, the AFRIMS respiratory laboratory is capable of performing molecular screening of 200 samples per week. Additionally, the field sites at the Kwai River Christian Hospital and in Kangphaeng Phet are each capable of screening an additional 100 samples per week, bringing the total capacity to 400 samples per week (AFRIMS, 2007b) (see Table 4-1).

In a periepidemic situation, AFRIMS would be able initially to alter the current testing algorithm to test for influenza A first and then, if positive,

TABLE 4-1 Summary of Surge Capability at AFRIMS

Condition	AFRIMS Respiratory Lab	Field Site × 2	Total Samples
Routine operation	200/week	200/week	400/week
Altered algorithm, influenza A and H5 first	300/week	300/week	600/week
Target only specific gene	1,000/week	1,000/week	2,000/week
24-hours-a-day, seven-days-a-week operations	3,000/week	2,000/week	5,000/week

SOURCE: AFRIMS, 2007b.

H5. This would allow screening of an additional 100 samples per week at the respiratory laboratory and an additional 50 per week at each field site, for a total of 600 samples per week.

Further refinement of the screening process, targeting only the gene required to rule in or out the strain of interest, would allow screening of up to 1.000 samples per week at the respiratory laboratory and 500 per week at each field site, for a total of 2,000 samples per week, without reassigning personnel. The limiting factor here would not be the laboratory, but data entry and quality assurance.

If required, AFRIMS could convert to a 24-hours–a-day, seven-days-a-week operation at the respiratory laboratory, thus trebling its sample processing capabilities. Such a surge would not be possible at the field sites, although a doubling of work hours is feasible. The best estimates of their short-term surge capabilities would be that the respiratory section could process 3,000 samples per week and each field site could process 1,000 samples per week, bringing AFRIMS's total molecular screening capabilities to 5,000 samples per week (AFRIMS, 2007b). This would require reassigning staff from other research activities and departments to maintain 24-hours-a-day, seven-days–a-week operations and would require equipment to be on stand-by in case of primary equipment failure. Additionally, AFRIMS does not stock enough reagents to accomplish these sample loads (nor would it be cost-effective), so reagents would have to be acquired quickly in order to carry out work at this volume.

Conclusions

AFRIMS has developed a plan and a chain of command to convert expendable research and other laboratory activities to support enhanced surveillance should human-to-human transmission by a novel avian influenza virus occur. More specifically, its plan describes how the lab will suspend certian activities and divert staff and resources to rapid around-the-clock PCR and diagnostic activities. This requires a limited amount of exposure of research staff to influenza work in order to train and prepare them. Included in this plan is the flexibility to send relevant staff to outbreak sites. In addition, AFRIMS's support of tabletop simulation exercises would help to identify areas of the national plans that need strengthening and direct future investments of pandemic preparedness funding in the region.

CAPACITY BUILDING

AFRIMS funded a significant number of capacity-building activities with the supplemental AI/PI funding from fiscal year 2006. The laboratory hired and trained core DoD-GEIS personnel to coordinate influenza surveillance at AFRIMS as well as laboratory and data entry personnel to work in the respiratory pathogen section in the department of virology. In addition, AFRIMS designed and awarded a contract to construct a BSL-3 laboratory facility. In order to improve its existing laboratory capacities, AFRIMS acquired real-time PCR and Mass Tag PCR technologies to perform respiratory pathogen identification as well as characterization and real-time PCR for the veterinary BSL-3 laboratory.

Virus culturing requires higher levels of biosafety because it produces higher concentrations of virus than are generally present in human nasal, throat, or other respiratory specimens. Importantly, culture is valuable because it affords greater capacity to characterize the virus and detect changes in antigenicity and nucleic acid sequences. These changes may further suggest that the virus is evolving to become more resistant to antiviral agents, more likely to cause severe disease, or more readily transmissible from human to human. Additionally, strains with similar sequences may be traced to a common origin, and this may suggest the source of infection. The design and construction of a BSL-3 laboratory is under way and expected to be completed by early 2008. The cost of this biosafety capacity is approximately $2 million, all of which comes from the supplemental funding.

The respiratory laboratory in Bangkok will have the capability for molecular diagnosis as well as subtyping strains to distinguish significant variants among the seasonal influenza isolates and to recognize strains that may emerge as candidate pandemic strains. An innovative capacity using mass tag spectroscopy to detect a wider range of respiratory pathogens, ranging from influenza to human metapneumovirus to mycoplasma, will be installed and evaluated in collaboration with a group at Columbia University. The viability of this technology is very much dependent on sound spectroscopy support. This venture may yield new information about pathogens that are currently unrecognized but that affect nationals, refugees, and military personnel alike. This respiratory laboratory will be greatly enhanced when the BSL-3 capacity is available for the virus isolation work.

As mentioned earlier, the major effort in Nepal involves WARUN, which has capacity for bacteriologic culture and will be fully functional in performing PCR assays for AI/PI by June 2007. In this effort a study will be conducted with the MoPH and several clinical sites looking at ILI. Specimens will be tested at the site of collection using rapid tests, and companion specimens will be transported to WARUN for PCR testing. The results will be confirmed at the AFRIMS laboratory in Bangkok and further characterized at AFIOH in San Antonio, Texas.

Training is an important element of the AFRIMS work, and it has been provided to U.S. embassies in the region as well as to public health agencies in Thailand, Nepal, and the Philippines; the training has covered such areas as specimen collection and transport, epidemiology, laboratory techniques, and AI recognition and response. In some cases the training sessions involved collaborations with other U.S. agencies or organizations within the countries where the training was conducted.

While in Kathmandu the site visit team met with the dean of the university's Institute of Medicine, himself a pediatrician, who expressed support for the DoD-GEIS-funded surveillance projects, emphasizing the importance of local technological understanding and improvements. The team saw great opportunities in Nepal to put into effect AFRIMS's skills as a WHO training center.

Conclusions

The IOM site visit team feels it a wise decision for AFRIMS to expand its diagnostic capabilities as this will allow it to culture H5N1 and other highly pathogenic strains of avian influenza virus as well as strains that may evolve or be recognized in the future. In conjunction with the expansion of the laboratory capabilities, AFRIMS will need to increase the number of trained personnel.

RECOMMENDATION 4-3. AFRIMS should continue to provide relevant training, including epidemiological training, to U.S. and local personnel to enable its expansion of laboratory capabilities.

COLLABORATION AND COORDINATION

AFRIMS collaborates on influenza virus surveillance with various organizations in Thailand as well as in the wider region (e.g. Nepal and the Philippines) and also has strong links with the Naval Medical Research Unit No. 2 (NAMRU-2) in Jakarta.

AFRIMS personnel are well aware of the importance of building trusting relationships with their partners and, as such, are careful and patient when establishing themselves in the various areas in which they work. In the interest of developing appropriate and sustainable projects, they work to find areas of mutual interest and aim to address the specific requests and needs of their partners. For example, the leadership understood that the ways in which it could assist the already established and fully functional influenza surveillance system of Thailand's MoPH were limited. The leadership therefore asked the MoPH what could be done to assist its efforts and, as a result, supported the development of the electronic reporting system for avian influenza.

Because AFRIMS is a relative newcomer in its AI/PI surveillance programs, relationships with organizations in the area doing similar work, such as U.S. Agency for International Development (USAID) and CDC, are also in their early stages of development. It is important to note, however, that these organizations are highly interested in future collaborations with AFRIMS. During the IOM team's meeting with the International Emerging Infections Program (IEIP), it was explained that two of the program's planned influenza studies intend to include a collaboration with AFRIMS. The team similarly heard during its meeting with representatives from USAID that increased interaction with AFRIMS is desired. It is believed that the completion of AFRIMS's BSL-3 laboratory will help to increase its collaborations with both existing partners and potential partners, such as IEIP. In addition, AFRIMS projects could also benefit from increased collaboration with personnel at DoD-GEIS headquarters to provide influenza-specific guidance and assistance.

The Nepal MoPH affirmed its relationship with WARUN and AFRIMS but noted that it expects to receive funding from the World Bank to build its own BSL-3. More specifically, the World Bank is giving Nepal $18 million, 60 percent of which will be allotted to the veterinary efforts and 40 percent to the human programs. When the IOM team visited WHO, officials there proposed to develop a model public health laboratory system in Nepal, working with the Nepal MoPH and personnel from AFRIMS/WARUN. This would require significant human resources input.

Conclusions

The support that AFRIMS provided for the Thai MoPH to develop a web-based reporting system should be a model for other AI/PI programs, and the development and use of similar systems in other countries or regions should be promoted. In an emergency there will be little opportunity to communicate critical information to those who need it most, and the web system will fill that void. The committee felt that Nepal would also benefit from AFRIMS's assistance in establishing a model system in Nepal for optimizing the delivery of regional and national public health laboratory services in collaboration with WHO and the Nepal MoPH.

The committee concluded that AFRIMS's ongoing collaboration with NAMRU-2 allows for improved utilization of AI/PI resources as well as redundant coverage for each of the laboratories in the event of a crisis (political, geologic, etc.) that might close one and not the other during a pandemic.

RECOMMENDATION 4-4. AFRIMS should continue to strengthen its relationship with NAMRU-2 in Indonesia and evaluate its roles in Asia and identify, where possible, critical geographic regions that are not covered by one or the other of these AI/PI programs.

REFERENCES

Air Force Institute for Operational Health (AFIOH). 2004. *DoD global influenza and other respiratory viral pathogens surveillance weekly update week 14 (4 Apr – 10 Apr)*. http://www.geis.fhp.osd.mil/GEIS/SurveillanceActivities/Influenza/Reports/influenza_2004-04-04.pdf (accessed September 5, 2007).

AFRIMS (Armed Forces Research Institute of Medical Sciences). 2007a. *AFRIMS influenza surveillance program—current and future* (unpublished).

AFRIMS. 2007b. *Estimated laboratory surge capacity* (unpublished).

AFRIMS. 2006. *AFRIMS human influenza isolate collection—current, prior to end FY07, and prior to end FY08* (unpublished).

Apisarnthanarak, A., R. Kitphati, K. Thongphubeth, P. Patoomanunt, P. Anthanont, W. Auwanit, P. Thawatsupha, M. Chittaganpitch, S. Saeng-Aroon, S. Waicharoen, P. Apisarnthanarak, G. A. Storch, L. M. Mundy, and V. J. Fraser. 2004. Atypical avian influenza (H5N1). *Emerging Infectious Diseases* 10(7):1321-1324.

DoD-GEIS (Department of Defense Global Emerging Infections System). 2007a. *Armed Forces Research Institute of Medical Sciences*. http://www.geis.fhp.osd.mil/GEIS/Training/AFRIMS.asp (accessed July 30, 2007).

DoD-GEIS. 2007b. *Department of Defense influenza surveillance sites worldwide, 2007* (unpublished).

Tiensin, T., P. Chaitaweesub, T. Songserm, A. Chaisingh, W. Hoonsuwan, C. Buranathai, T. Parakamawongsa, S. Premashthira, A. Amonsin, M. Gilbert, M. Nielen, and A. Stegeman. 2005. Highly pathogenic avian influenza H5N1, Thailand, 2004. *Emerging Infectious Diseases* 11(11):1664-1672.

WHO (World Health Organization). 2004. *Avian influenza—situation in Thailand*. http://www.who.int/csr/don/2004_09_28a/en/print.html (accessed June 12, 2007).

WHO. 2007a. *H5N1 avian influenza: Timeline of major events*. http://www.who.int/csr/disease/avian_influenza/Timeline_2007_03_20.pdf (accessed July 30, 2007).

WHO. 2007b. *Cumulative number of confirmed human cases of avian influenza A/(H5N1) reported to WHO*. http://www.who.int/csr/disease/avian_influenza/country/cases_table_2007_07_25/en/index.html (accessed July 30, 2007).

WHO. 2007c. *Avian influenza outbreaks in South-East Asia*. http://www.searo.who.int/EN/section10/section1027.htm (accessed June 12, 2007).

LIST OF CONTACTS

DoD-GEIS AFRIMS Assessment: Thailand

Rodney Coldren, GEIS Director, Armed Forces Research Institute of Medical Sciences, Bangkok, Thailand
Robert V. Gibbons, Department of Virology, Armed Forces Research Institute of Medical Sciences, Bangkok, Thailand
Richard Jarman, Department of Virology, Armed Forces Research Institute of Medical Sciences, Bangkok, Thailand
Khir Saw Aye Myint, Department of Virology, Armed Forces Research Institute of Medical Sciences, Bangkok, Thailand
Bonnie Smoak, Commander, US Army Medical Component, Armed Forces Research Institute of Medical Sciences, Bangkok, Thailand
Bryan Sweeney, Influenza Program Manager, Armed Forces Research Institute of Medical Sciences, Bangkok, Thailand
In-Kyu Yoon, Department of Virology, Armed Forces Research Institute of Medical Sciences, Bangkok, Thailand
Jim Waller, Economic Section, Embassy of the United States, Bangkok, Thailand
Sudarat Damrongwatanapokin, Regional Development Mission, Asia/ United States Agency for International Development, Bangkok, Thailand
Susan Maloney, Division of Global Migration and Quarantine, Centers for Disease Control and Prevention, Atlanta, Georgia
Henry Baggett, International Emerging Infections Program, Centers for Disease Control and Prevention/Thailand Ministry of Public Health, Nonthaburi, Thailand
Leonard F. Peruski, International Emerging Infections Program, Centers for Disease Control and Prevention/Thailand Ministry of Public Health, Nonthaburi, Thailand
Wiwan Sanasuttipun, International Emerging Infections Program, Centers for Disease Control and Prevention/Thailand Ministry of Public Health, Nonthaburi, Thailand
Somsak Thamthitiwat, International Emerging Infections Program, Centers for Disease Control and Prevention/Thailand Ministry of Public Health, Nonthaburi, Thailand
Malinee Chittaganpitch, National Institutes of Health, Bangkok, Thailand
Rungrueng Kitphati, National Institutes of Health, Bangkok, Thailand
Krongraew Supawat, National Institutes of Health, Bangkok, Thailand

DoD-GEIS WARUN Assessment: Nepal

Sanjaya Kr. Shrestha, Walter Reed AFRIMS Research Unit Nepal, Kathmandu, Nepal
Mrigendra Pd. Shrestha, Walter Reed AFRIMS Research Unit Nepal, Kathmandu, Nepal
Ruthanne Taylor, U.S. Embassy Medical Unit Chief, American Embassy, Kathmandu, Nepal
James F. Moriarty, U.S. Ambassador to Nepal, Kathmandu, Nepal
Scott Taylor, Defense Attaché, American Embassy, Kathmandu, Nepal
Ramesh K. Adinkani, Institute of Medicine, Kathmandu, Nepal
Manas Kumar Banerjee, Epidemiology and Disease Control Division of Department of Health Services, Kathmandu, Nepal
Sarala Malla, Ministry of Health and Population, Department of Health Services, National Public Health Laboratory, Kathmandu, Nepal
Jeetendra Man Shrestha, Epidemiology and Disease Control Division of Department of Health Services, Kathmandu, Nepal
Sailesh B. Pradhan, Kathmandu Medical College Teaching Hospital, Kathmandu, Nepal
Manohar Prasad Gupta, Tribhuvan University Teaching Hospital, Kathmandu, Nepal
Yagya Laxmi Shakya, Tribhuvan University Teaching Hospital, Kathmandu, Nepal
Prativa Pandey, CIWEC Clinical Travel Medicine Center, Kathmandu, Nepal
Margarita Ronderos, World Health Organization Country Office for Nepal, Kathmandu, Nepal
Kan Tun, World Health Organization Country Office for Nepal, Kathmandu, Nepal
Prakash Ghimire, Programme for Immunization of Preventable Diseases, World Health Organization, Kathmandu, Nepal

SCHEDULE OF EVENTS
DoD-GEIS AFRIMS and WARUN Assessments

Bangkok, Thailand and Kathmandu, Nepal
Participants: Mary J. R. Gilchrist
Kennedy Francis Shortridge
Kimberly Weingarten
March 12–17, 2007

Monday, March 12, 2007

0830-0930	**In-brief at Vet Med building** Col. Smoak Lt. Col. Coldren Mr. Sweeney
0930-1030	**Overview of GEIS program**
1030-1045	Break
1045-1130	**Briefing on BSL-3**
1130-1215	Lunch
1215-1330	**Tour of AFRIMS main building**
1330-1345	Return to Vet Med
1345-1445	**Overview of Department of Immunology and Medicine avian influenza program**
1445-1545	**Overview of RTA influenza surveillance** Enterics department
1545-1615	**Briefing on Department of Veterinary Medicine**
1615-1700	**Tour of Vet Med and BSL-3 suite construction site**
1700-1730	Return to hotel

Tuesday, March 13, 2007

0800-1000	**Briefing on Department of Virology**
1000-1015	Break
1015-1145	**Meeting with USAID personnel and state department science and tech officer**
1145-1230	Lunch
1230-1315	Travel to Ministry of Public Health (MoPH)
1315-1445	**Meeting with IEIP staff and MoPH representatives**
1445-1500	Break
1500-1645	**Continued discussions with MoPH representatives**
1645-1745	Return to hotel

Wednesday, March 14, 2007

0730-1330	Fly to Kathmandu, Nepal
1400-1530	**Facility tour and staff introductions**
1530-1630	**Presentation on WARUN activities** Dr. Sanjaya Kr. Shrestha, Head of Station, WARUN
1600-1630	Return to hotel

Thursday, March 15, 2007

0900-1030	**Discussion of purpose of visit and importance of influenza surveillance program** Mr. James F. Moriarty, U.S. ambassador to Nepal Lt. Col. Scott Taylor, defense attache Dr. Ruthanne Taylor, U.S. embassy medical unit chief
1030-1130	**Discussion of purpose of visit, the influenza diagnostic support program, and future plans of the Department of Health Services** Dr. Manas Kumar Banerjee, Director of EDCD Dr. Jeetendra Man Shrestha, avian influenza coordinator of EDCD Dr. Margarita Ronderos, WHO medical officer and UN influenza coordinator
1430-1550	**Discussion of veterinary laboratory work** Dr. Rebati Man Shrestha, director of Central Veterinary Laboratory
1550-1630	**Meeting about construction plans for laboratory** Dr. Kan Tun, country representative to WHO Dr. Margarita Ronderos
1630-1700	Return to hotel

Friday, March 16, 2007

1100-1600	**Visit sentinel influenza sites** (**TUTH, CIWEC, KMC, BDRC**)
1600-1630	Return to hotel

Saturday, March 17, 2007

0900-1100	**De-brief**
1100-1200	Lunch
1200-1800	Departure

5

Naval Medical Research Unit 3 Egypt Avian and Pandemic Influenza Activities

U.S. Naval Medical Research Unit No. 3 (NAMRU-3) is a U.S. Navy research biosafety level 3 enhanced (BSL-3E) laboratory with extensive human and animal viral diagnostic capacity located in Cairo, Egypt. NAMRU-3 is one of the largest medical research laboratories in the North Africa-Middle East region and is also the regional influenza reference laboratory for the Eastern Mediterranean Regional Office (EMRO) of the World Health Organization (WHO) with close ties to the influenza laboratory at the U.S. Centers for Disease Control and Prevention (CDC) (DoD-GEIS, 2007a).

NAMRU-3 was formally established by the U.S. Secretary of the Navy in 1946 at the site of the former Typhus Commission in Cairo, Egypt (IOM, 2001; DoD-GEIS, 2007a). The early work at NAMRU-3 focused, in collaboration with the Egyptian Ministry of Health, on rickettsial diseases and febrile diseases (smallpox, meningitis, etc.) in patients admitted to the adjacent Abbasia Fever Hospital, Egypt's largest fever hospital (DoD-GEIS, 2007a). In addition, NAMRU-3 has been heavily involved in avian and pandemic influenza surveillance. Though NAMRU-3 has historically been dedicated to a laboratory- and field-based infectious-disease research mission, influenza surveillance activities have been conducted at NAMRU-3 since the 1999 initiation of funding from the Department of Defense Global Emerging Infections Surveillance and Response System (DoD-GEIS) for seasonal influenza surveillance activities.

DoD-GEIS support for NAMRU-3 influenza surveillance and response projects totaled $4 million in fiscal year 2006. Using these funds, NAMRU-

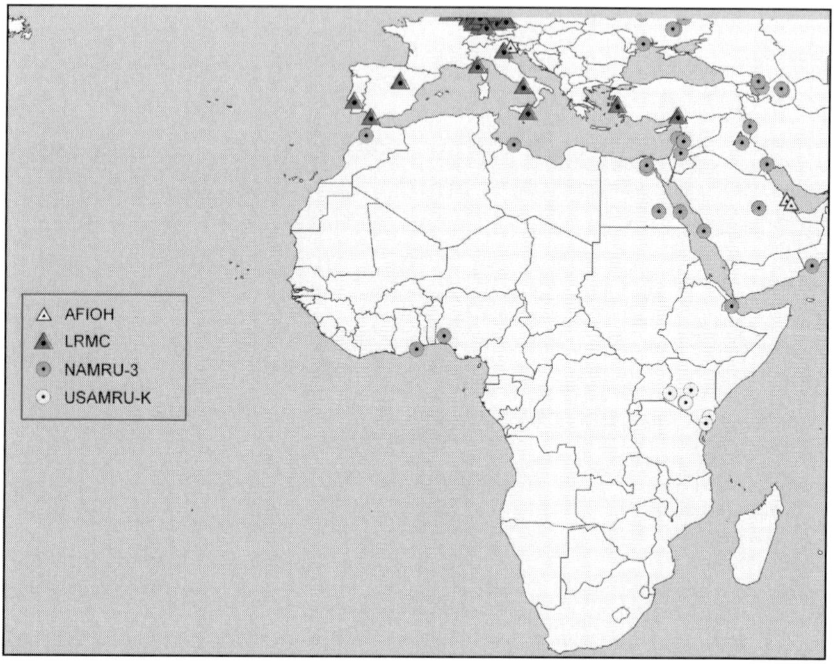

FIGURE 5-1 DoD's regional presence in influenza surveillance (Africa), 2007.
SOURCE: DoD-GEIS, 2007b.

3 expanded a number of its activities, such as conducting training on influenza diagnosis, helping to build national influenza laboratory capacity in Egypt and the region (including Afghanistan, Jordan, Libya, and Ghana), and assisting with the WHO global influenza surveillance program through bilateral and trilateral influenza surveillance projects (see Figure 5-1). Limited migratory bird surveillance is also being conducted using DoD-GEIS funds. This surveillance has become more robust with the addition of avian influenza/pandemic influenza (AI/PI) funding from DoD-GEIS.

A site visit team of the Institute of Medicine (IOM) Committee for the Assessment of DoD-GEIS Influenza Surveillance and Response Programs visited NAMRU-3 from March 4-9, 2007.[1] A list of the people with whom the site visit team met and the itinerary that was followed can be found at the end of this chapter.

---

[1]Prior to the committee's visit to NAMRU-3, the laboratory staff provided the committee with detailed background information on NAMRU-3 and the pandemic/avian influenza activities it was supporting. These materials are available from the IOM in the Public Access File.

INFLUENZA IN EGYPT

The first confirmation of H5N1 in Egypt was made in February 2006 (WHO, 2007a). At that time, seven outbreaks of avian influenza (AI) virus subtype H5N1 were reported throughout seven governorates in Egypt (Cairo, Giza, Menia, Qina, Kalyubeya, Behera, and Dakahlia) (USDA, 2006). These outbreaks were diagnosed by the Animal Health Research Institute, Egypt's national laboratory, and confirmed as H5N1 by NAMRU-3 (OIE, 2006). Reports of outbreaks continued to be received until December 2006 (WHO, 2007a).

In addition to the poultry outbreaks affecting both backyard and commercial poultry, Egypt has had 36 human cases of avian influenza infection, the highest number of bird flu cases among humans outside of Asia. Of these 36 cases, 15 have resulted in death (WHO, 2007b). Though avian influenza has been found in several areas of Africa, Egypt is one of only two African countries—the other being Nigeria—to have reported a human case of the infection (WHO, 2007a).

MANAGEMENT AND PLANNING

Generally, DoD-GEIS activities at NAMRU-3 are coordinated by the director of the Research Sciences Department and carried out by other research departments, including virology research, disease surveillance, enteric disease research, and vector biology research. DoD-GEIS AI/PI supplemental funding is managed primarily by the virology program head.

It is reportedly challenging to manage the large sums of money related to AI/PI activities, especially when the financing arrives late in the fiscal year, although in fiscal year 2006, when NAMRU-3 staff had to receive and obligate funds and then implement projects in a short period of time, they proved flexible enough to do so. In the future, additional personnel in both the finance and supply departments would potentially help to streamline the acquisition of equipment and reagents, but in 2006 the major delay was due to external circumstances. The purchase of high-dollar equipment or initiation of contracts must be routed through the Fleet and Industrial Supply Center (FISC). NAMRU-3 experienced up to a six-month delay when purchasing equipment since FISC did not award many contracts until September 2006 even though the purchase requests were submitted in April of that year.

Staffing

All of the research departments at NAMRU-3 have a variety of ongoing projects, only some of which are AI/PI-related. There are no dedicated

DoD-GEIS personnel. However, the AI supplemental funding is being used to support 22 persons associated with 18 full-time equivalent (FTE) positions. These personnel include two virologists, three molecular biologists, two medical epidemiologists, four laboratory technologists, and two data clerks. The NAMRU-3 has supported a variety of employees with the supplemental funding, including a number of U.S. Government Service employees, non-personnel service contractors, and locally employed staff (Egyptian nationals). As the capacity of the laboratory increases, NAMRU-3 would like to hire additional laboratory technologists in the areas of viral isolation and molecular biology.

While there is still great need at the laboratory for expanded epidemiological expertise, with the increased personnel from CDC's global disease detection and response program NAMRU-3 expects that these deficits will be covered. At the time of the IOM team's site visit, it was still unclear what role the CDC staff would play at the laboratory, and a memorandum of understanding regarding the exact nature of tasks and activities that CDC will perform had not yet been written.

Given the importance of its geopolitical location in the Middle East, one of NAMRU-3's greatest strengths is its reliance on Foreign Service Nationals to play key roles in the management and activities of the laboratory. NAMRU-3 has used this strength in expanding its avian/pandemic influenza programs and broadening its laboratory capacity, thus strengthening activities for the countries in the EMRO region.

Technology and Information Management

The technology capabilities of NAMRU-3 were found to be substantial and more than adequate to manage the current increase in activity resulting from additional AI funding. At the moment, NAMRU-3 relies on informal information-sharing methods to provide status reports to relevant government officials. While these methods do serve to strengthen personal relationships between NAMRU-3 staff and government officials, if human-to-human transmission occurs these informal channels will not be sufficient to provide timely and accurate information early in a pandemic. As more cases of avian influenza are identified in Egypt and the region, it will become increasingly important for key laboratory network hubs like NAMRU-3 to have formal systems in place to share information at the local, regional, and global levels in an accurate and timely way. Various sources of information, including findings from human surveillance, avian surveillance, and outbreak investigations, will have to be coordinated and shared with the relevant governments and with the international agencies involved in setting policy and implementing prevention and intervention efforts.

One mechanism that NAMRU-3 is using to share relevant information in the country and the region is the production of a weekly bulletin on the influenza situation in the Middle East. While these bulletins are currently very useful, NAMRU-3—in conjunction with the host governments, EMRO, and WHO headquarters—will need to develop a real-time system if human-to-human transmission occurs.

Conclusions

The site visit team noted that the planning and implementation of specific projects being conducted by NAMRU-3 were well executed but the organizational strategy needed to guide the laboratory's future influenza activities is lacking. NAMRU-3 staff were planning to hold a meeting regarding the laboratory's organizational direction and how NAMRU-3 can best meet the needs of countries in the region.

RECOMMENDATION 5-1. NAMRU-3 should prepare a short-term (2-3 years) strategic plan that identifies its priorities (surveillance/research and implementation/service delivery) in the AI/PI program and indicates NAMRU-3's role in the prepandemic stage.

The staffing is acceptable for the current activities, but NAMRU-3 may need to make staffing and equipment adjustments when it moves into the early pandemic phase. For example, staff members from other units may be cross-trained and deployed to assist with enhanced surveillance when their research activities are no longer a priority, due to the emergency.

NAMRU-3 staff members suggest that their method of information sharing—making telephone calls to pertinent local and international offices in order of priority—is adequate. It may not be adequate, however, in the case of an outbreak of pandemic influenza. The committee concluded that the development of the manual system as well as a web-based, password-protected reporting system would benefit NAMRU-3 and the host countries with which it works. Redundancy in reporting systems may also be useful. Radio, telephone, web and satellite communications are all vulnerable to breakdown due to overuse.

In a pandemic phase, all of the data being produced by NAMRU-3 would ideally be available on a protected website for partners like WHO and the Ministry of Health. Avian influenza data could be linked with the infectious disease database managed by the Ministry of Health. NAMRU-3 should develop an improved system of communication that enables all qualified partners to access information without reliance on individual phone or e-mail communication, such as a protected website or blast fax system.

RECOMMENDATION 5-2. NAMRU-3 should develop and implement a comprehensive information-management system as soon as possible in order to prepare for the expanded needs that will be present during a potential pandemic and to improve routine information sharing in the EMRO region.

SURVEILLANCE

NAMRU-3 has greatly contributed to the avian influenza surveillance effort in Egypt and the Middle East. While most of its activities focusing on human influenza surveillance are related to building the capacity of national influenza centers, NAMRU-3 is participating in a targeted project for U.S. military personnel. In addition, NAMRU-3 is working with the Ministry of Environment in Egypt and its sister DoD laboratory, the U.S. Army Medical Research Unit- Kenya (USAMRU-K), to conduct surveillance of migratory birds.

Human Surveillance

Both independently and in its role as a WHO collaborating center, NAMRU-3 works to strengthen national laboratory capacity and also functions as a reference laboratory for countries across the region. In its effort to make best use of the supplemental funding for AI/PI influenza and strengthen the regional influenza network, NAMRU-3 has focused most of its funding for human influenza surveillance on providing support equipment and technical assistance to national influenza laboratories in places like Egypt, Afghanistan, Syria, Pakistan, Oman, Saudi Arabia, and Morocco (NAMRU-3, 2007b) (see Figure 5-2). Through these capacity-building activities, NAMRU-3 hopes to expand the regional surveillance network and establish a flow of influenza data and isolates from countries previously not represented in this network. Additional information is provided in the Capacity section below.

One primary benefit to the capacity-building efforts of NAMRU-3 is access to influenza samples and isolates from across the region. While NAMRU-3 is not collecting samples directly, researchers at NAMRU-3, working through partner governments' laboratory systems and previously established seasonal influenza sites, are able to analyze samples from across the region and to provide that information to U.S. agencies like the CDC and to multilateral coordinators like the Food and Agricultural Organization (FAO) and WHO.

Between July 2006 and January 2007, NAMRU-3 received 2,470 samples from its seasonal influenza and H5 referencing activities, of which it processed 2006 (NAMRU-3, 2007c). These samples came from 11 coun-

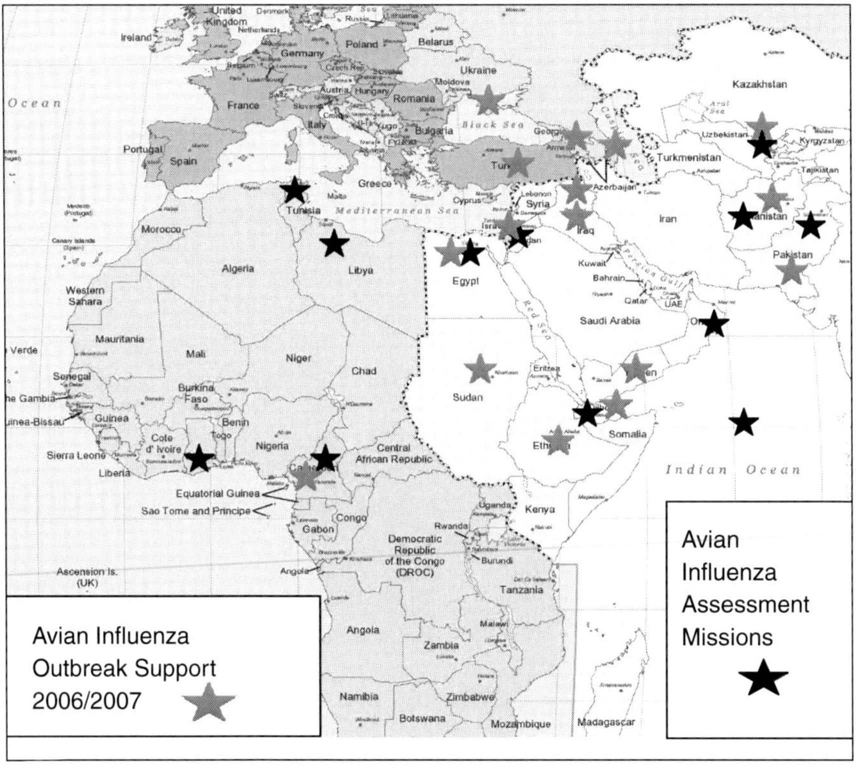

FIGURE 5-2 NAMRU-3 avian influenza assessment missions and outbreak support.
SOURCE: NAMRU-3, 2007b.

tries in the EMRO region plus Nigeria, with the majority of samples coming from NAMRU-3's host country, Egypt. Fifty-one of the samples received were sent to NAMRU-3 for H5 reference testing by laboratories in Egypt, Iraq, Yemen, and Afghanistan; 22 of these samples were processed, resulting in four positive results for H5N1 (NAMRU-3, 2007c). All the samples positive for influenza H5N1 were from Egypt.

NAMRU-3 has also contributed to the development and implementation of an influenza-related surveillance project managed out of Doha, Qatar, looking at respiratory disease in active-duty U.S. military populations. A satellite laboratory allows for the collection of respiratory samples from troops on rest and recuperation from Afghanistan and Iraq. NAMRU-3 has also provided reference support to diagnose respiratory diseases among troops deployed in Iraq and at Camp Arifjan, Kuwait.

Animal Surveillance

NAMRU-3 supports avian influenza surveillance in migratory birds in Ukraine, Egypt, and Kenya. NAMRU-3's location in Egypt provides a unique opportunity to collect specimens and identify isolates from migratory birds traveling from Europe through the Egyptian flyways to sub-Saharan Africa. In addition, NAMRU-3 acts as a reference laboratory in the EMRO region for other suspected H5N1 animal cases.

In Egypt, NAMRU-3's migratory bird surveillance is conducted in collaboration with the Ministry of Environment throughout the Nile Delta region, as this is a major location for stopover of migratory birds during their transit. Current environmental ministry collection sites are Port Said (Rasheed), El-Sharkeya, El-Manzala, Port Fouad, El-Fayoum, El-Arish, Sharm El-Sheik, Aswan, El-Minya, Alexandria, and Domietta. NAMRU-3 and the MoE have provided active surveillance of wild migratory birds since October 2003 in an effort to detect circulating influenza viruses. Specimens are collected using the appropriate personal protective equipment. Specimens such as tracheal swabs, cloacal swabs, tissue, serum, and so on are collected based on the method performed. As a result of these activities in Egypt, NAMRU-3 received and processed 490 wild bird samples in January 2007. Of these 48 (9.8 percent) tested positive for influenza A, 2 (0.3 percent) tested positive for H5, and none were found to be positive for H5N1 (NAMRU-3, 2007c).

NAMRU-3 has established similar surveillance activities in Kenya and Ukraine. As a result of NAMRU-3's ongoing migratory bird surveillance activities in Ukraine, it was able to confirm an H5N1 highly pathogenic avian influenza outbreak among migratory birds in February 2006.

Through its animal H5 reference testing, NAMRU-3 was the first laboratory to diagnose and confirm influenza H5N1 infections in poultry in Afghanistan, Djibouti, Egypt, Iraq, Jordan, and Kazakhstan. Between July 2006 and January 2007, NAMRU-3 received 51 animal samples for H5 reference testing. Of the 46 which were processed by NAMRU-3, nine samples, most of which came from chickens and doves found dead, were found positive for influenza H5N1.

Conclusions

While NAMRU-3 is not conducting any human surveillance activities itself, the committee found that NAMRU-3 is an integral advisor to host country government in development of its surveillance programs and the associated laboratory capacity. As the regional surveillance network expands, the committee feels it would be beneficial to expand diagnostics to include emerging influenza pathogens beyond H5N1 as well as to integrate seasonal influenza and AI/PI programs as much as possible.

RECOMMENDATION 5-3. NAMRU-3 should assist the host country to develop the capacity to find emerging influenza pathogens beyond H5N1 and should integrate seasonal influenza and AI/PI programs as much as possible.

In terms of avian surveillance, the committee found that NAMRU-3 is working successfully with the Ministry of Environment to conduct influenza surveillance on wild bird populations in Egypt. However, NAMRU-3 does not conduct routine surveillance on domestic bird or poultry populations in Egypt. The Ministry of Agriculture reportedly does conduct surveillance at sites of previous H5N1 infection or sites of major poultry production, but little information on these activities was available.

RECOMMENDATION 5-4. NAMRU-3 should explore opportunities to support the Ministry of Agriculture in increasing surveillance of domestic birds kept in homes and back yards.

LABORATORY

NAMRU-3 headquarters in Cairo, Egypt, has extensive laboratory capacities, particularly in virology (DoD-GEIS, 2007a). The NAMRU-3 campus houses two BSL-3 laboratories. Using DoD-GEIS supplemental funding, NAMRU-3 has been able to increase the laboratory capacity at its headquarters, including equipment, reagents, BSL-3 space, reverse transcription polymerase chain reaction (RT-PCR) capability, and personnel (NAMRU-3, 2007b). NAMRU-3's H5 surveillance sample testing is based mainly on RT-PCR methodology. NAMRU-3's mobile laboratory response capability has been increased by the addition of four mobile RT-PCR devices, which have enhanced both its ability to address multiple outbreaks concurrently and to perform training at external sites. NAMRU-3 currently has the laboratory capability to do subtyping for influenza A, H5, H9 and N1 by RT-PCR; influenza A by ELISA; and H1, H16 and B by HI assays.

NAMRU-3 has also identified four satellite laboratories in Libya, Jordan, Ghana, and Afghanistan in which it plans to expand diagnostic capacity, both to strengthen this capacity closer to the bulk of U.S. troops in the region and to expand the regional surveillance network (NAMRU-3, 2007b). These NAMRU-3-established satellite laboratories will soon have the capacity for virus isolation and molecular identification of respiratory viruses. NAMRU-3 is working to increase the capacity of these laboratories though the acquisition of incubators, light cyclers, -80°C freezers, centrifuges, and other necessary supplies and equipment.

While NAMRU-3 is not leading any avian influenza surveillance activities, the NAMRU-3 laboratory is currently participating at various levels in the testing of samples and the isolation of virus from avian influenza surveillance systems across the EMRO region and beyond. The laboratory system used for influenza surveillance in the EMRO region is quite centralized. Laboratories located outside the capital cities have very limited capacity and thus are relegated solely to collecting specimens; some central labs are still working to develop the needed capability to process avian influenza samples. Because of NAMRU-3's status as a WHO collaborating center, the laboratory has a different role from some other DoD-GEIS laboratories with regard to avian influenza surveillance. For example, in Egypt NAMRU-3 is currently acting as the Ministry of Health's quality assurance mechanism. Possible AI samples are confirmed by NAMRU-3 after being sent to the central laboratory from identified fever and chest hospitals. In other countries, such as Libya, Jordan, Ghana, and Afghanistan, NAMRU-3 is still doing primary screening while these countries work to establish national laboratories with PCR capabilities. For suspected cases of AI in humans, NAMRU-3 turns around samples on the same day, while for seasonal flu virus isolation and subtyping the turnaround time is approximately 2 weeks. Results are reported to the Ministry of Health, WHO, NAMRU-3, and other influenza partners as appropriate (DoD-GEIS, the Naval Medical Research Center, CDC, and so on).

In Egypt, the Ministry of Agriculture processes all of the domestic and poultry specimens at its central laboratory in Cairo. Although the Ministry of Agriculture and the Ministry of Health have real-time RT-PCR capacity, the Ministry of Environment has NAMRU-3 do the primary screening of wild bird samples under an active surveillance program funded by DoD-GEIS because it does not have the needed PCR capabilities. NAMRU-3 reports to the Ministry of Environment on migratory bird surveillance specimens within 10 days of submission. NAMRU-3 also does the primary screening of wild bird samples for its other collaborative wild bird surveillance sites, including samples sent to Egypt from NAMRU-3's sister laboratory, USAMRU-K.

Conclusions

NAMRU-3 facilities play an essential role in supporting influenza surveillance in Egypt and the region. Because of the laboratory's unique position, NAMRU-3 has an opportunity to contribute to the knowledge of specific viral and bacterial agents in respiratory disease and should consider the purchase of multiplex diagnostic equipment in order to simplify quality control, increase automation, and expand the laboratory's ability to detect a broad array of etiologic agents.

RECOMMENDATION 5-5. NAMRU-3 should explore the expansion of laboratory capacity to include multiplex diagnostic equipment for respiratory diseases.

At the current time NAMRU-3's laboratory facilities are adequate for its influenza activities. However, as the number of avian influenza cases increases, changes will have to be made to the regular operations of the laboratory. In the days, weeks, or months before a pandemic takes over completely, laboratory testing that is rapid and accurate will help to diminish panic if it can rule out the pandemic strain where possible and rule in the pandemic strain where necessary. Planning out a move to a response mode in advance will be critical. The committee concluded that determining what equipment would be needed to increase laboratory output on a per-FTE basis—e.g. automated extraction, additional real-time PCR, and redundancy in sequencing devices if considered critical—will be central to NAMRU-3's ability to handle an increase in samples. Instead of expanding laboratory staffing, automation might be increased to optimize the throughput and the speed of processing. For example, automated extraction devices, which have throughput similar to that of real-time PCR instruments, would increase the capacity of the laboratory without necessarily increasing the laboratory staff. In addition, while NAMRU-3's research is valuable, justified, and leads to good information, a significant portion could be suspended in the case of a pandemic.

RECOMMENDATION 5-6. NAMRU-3 should develop a plan to expand its laboratory capacity in an early pandemic phase based on an assessment of how instrumentation and cross-training can be employed to optimize the laboratory and move from moderate throughput to high throughput with minimal staffing changes.

RESPONSE CAPACITY

NAMRU-3 has two primary response capacity functions. First, since it serves as a reference or quality control laboratory for many of the national central laboratories in the EMRO region, it has been called upon to provide surge capacity when the number of either human or animal samples exceeds the capacity of national laboratories. Second, NAMRU-3 has often been called on by WHO or national ministries of health to participate in outbreak-response teams (NAMRU-3, 2007b) (see Figure 5.2).

Outbreak Response

Avian influenza outbreak response requires portable PCR capacity, appropriate personal protective equipment, adequate supplies, reagents, and a diverse mix of staff. Using DoD-GEIS AI supplemental funding, NAMRU-3 has been able to increase its outbreak-response capability with regards to equipment, reagents, and personnel (NAMRU-3, 2007b). The four additional mobile real-time PCR machines have greatly enhanced its ability to simultaneously deploy to multiple sites to assist in outbreak response. Currently, NAMRU-3 has the capacity to field up to four teams simultaneously to support forward outbreak response. Teams are generally made up of a laboratorian, epidemiologist, and a veterinarian.

In the past six months, NAMRU-3 has conducted respiratory disease outbreak investigations in humans and poultry in Kazakhstan (confirmed H5N1), Ukraine (confirmed H5N1), Iraq (H9), Yemen (Newcastle disease) and Ethiopia (non-AI) (NAMRU-3, 2007b). To date, no human samples tested have been positive for avian influenza. Field teams have deployed with personal protective equipment, ruggedized light cyclers, reagents, and supplies. Teams have performed field and laboratory necropsies on poultry and done testing for avian and human influenza. In addition to providing diagnostic support, NAMRU-3 provided training on the proper sampling, handling, and diagnosis of avian influenza.

NAMRU-3 reported not being able to meet all of the requests it is currently receiving for outbreak response or assistance. To meet the regional needs for assistance and respond to outbreaks, NAMRU-3 has found it necessary to give priority to certain requests, such as those with the greatest risk of H5N1 and those with new data or isolates. This prioritization helps the laboratory staff to balance its commitment to rapid deployment to outbreaks occurring simultaneously in different regions with its commitment to maintaining assessment and training capacity.

Surge Capacity

Because of its role as a WHO collaborating center, NAMRU-3 will extend its functions beyond outbreak response in the next influenza pandemic. As has occurred in the past, NAMRU-3 will be called upon to provide surge capacity as the number of possible pandemic influenza samples increases.

For routine operations—normal workdays over a five day work week by current virology program personnel—NAMRU-3 estimated it would be able to process 450 specimens per week at the headquarters in Cairo using molecular diagnostics on any of multiple ABI 7300/7500 systems and targeting A, H5, and N1 genes along with an RNP (internal human RNA

TABLE 5-1 Summary of Surge Capability at NAMRU-3—Routine Operations

Condition	NAMRU-3	Field Sites × 4	Total Samples
Molecular Diagnostics	450 specimens/ week	450 specimens/ week	2,250 specimens/ week
Sequencing	60 specimens/week	0	60 specimens/ week
Culture (SPF & MDCK)	30 specimens/week	0	30 specimens/ week
Microneutralization	50 specimens/week	0	50 specimens/ week
Antiviral Susceptibility	300 specimens/week	0	300 specimens/ week

SOURCE: NAMRU-3, 2007a.

control) gene. NAMRU-3 also estimated that the DoD-GEIS field sites in Afghanistan, Jordan, Libya, and Ghana could function at 450 specimens per week if needed (NAMRU-3, 2007a) (see Table 5-1).

If the testing algorithm were altered to first test for influenza A and then, if positive, to test for H5, NAMRU-3 did not expect that the decrease in gene targets would lead to a corresponding increase in the number of tests that could be performed because the rate-limiting step is RNA extraction, which runs at 24 samples per person per hood over a two-hour period (see Table 5-2). NAMRU-3 did say that in order to increase the overall number of extractions performed per day—thereby increasing its weekly in-house throughput—it would require the laboratory to allocate four personnel to each of four molecular diagnostic biological safety cabinets to perform RNA extractions.

TABLE 5-2 Summary of Surge Capability at NAMRU-3—Altered Algorithm (Influenza A and H5 first)

Condition	NAMRU-3	Field Sites × 4	Total Samples
Molecular Diagnostics	1,600 specimens/ week	450 specimens/ week	3,400 specimens/ week
Sequencing	60 specimens/ week	0	60 specimens/week
Culture (SPF & MDCK)	30 specimens/ week	0	30 specimens/week
Microneutralization	50 specimens/ week	0	50 specimens/week
Antiviral Susceptibility	300 specimens/ week	0	300 specimens/week

SOURCE: NAMRU-3, 2007a.

Because NAMRU-3 receives WHO and courier shipments, it is expected that the number of specimens arriving daily would vary (e.g., 200 specimens one day, 750 another, and so on). During surge efforts NAMRU-3 would deal with the specimens received using a first in/first out rule.

Under the scenario of working 24 hours a day, seven days a week, the virology program would divert molecular diagnostic personnel from all of the programs at NAMRU-3. Virology has seven personnel competent in molecular diagnostics. Six personnel from enterics, three from disease surveillance, and one from vector biology have been given formal training on influenza diagnostics or are competent in molecular techniques such as RNA extraction, or both.

Four individuals would be performing extractions at all times while one person would begin real-time runs on selected gene targets, which adds up to a requirement of five molecular diagnostics personnel required per 9-hour shift, with some overlap. Each individual would extract approximately 90 specimens over a 9-hour shift. Thus the best case scenario is 360 specimens per shift, 1,080 specimens per day, or 7,560 specimens per week at NAMRU-3. This estimate was reduced by NAMRU-3 to 7,000 specimens per week in order to anticipate transitional delays (see Table 5-3).

The laboratory components of NAMRU-3's outbreak response teams use the 32-well format mobile RT-PCR machine. To maintain quality control and assurance, as well as biosafety, it would not be advisable to have the single laboratorian run more than 150 specimens (five runs, 30 specimens per run, plus controls) per day (see Table 5-4). Furthermore, deploying forward laboratory support will eliminate one molecular biologist from NAMRU-3, thereby requiring additional consideration in terms of staffing.

TABLE 5-3 Summary of Surge Capability at NAMRU-3—24-Hours-a-Day, Seven-Days-a-Week Operations and Altered Algorithm (Influenza A and H5 first)

Condition	NAMRU-3	Field Sites × 4	Total Samples
Molecular Diagnostics	7,000 specimens/ week	450 specimens/week	8,800 specimens/week
Sequencing	160 specimens/ week	0	160 specimens/week
Culture (SPF & MDCK)	210 specimens/ week	0	210 specimens/week
Microneutralization	500 specimens/ week	0	500 specimens/week
Antiviral Susceptibility	1,050 specimens/ week	0	1,050 specimens/week

SOURCE: NAMRU-3, 2007a.

TABLE 5-4 Summary of Surge Capability at NAMRU-3—Outbreak Support

Condition	NAMRU-3	Field Sites × 4	Total Samples
Molecular Diagnostics	1,050 specimens/ week	0	1,050 specimens/ week

SOURCE: NAMRU-3, 2007a.

It should also be mentioned that a deployed team is limited in terms of total specimens it can test, based on local storage facilities and space constraints. It is likely that testing 1,000 total specimens run by a deployed team is approaching the maximum. A total of 500 specimens is more feasible during one deployment period.

Conclusions

In terms of laboratory diagnosis, field investigation, and collaboration (e.g., with the Egyptian Ministry of Health and Population and the WHO), NAMRU-3 is well situated to respond to infectious disease outbreaks such as avian influenza in the region. The DoD-GEIS AI/PI funding has enhanced and strengthened the unique regional capacity of NAMRU-3. However, in an early influenza pandemic, NAMRU-3 will most likely be needed to provide both outbreak response and laboratory surge capacity simultaneously. For these activities its laboratory capacity will need to be expanded. NAMRU-3 has sufficiently strengthened its mobile outbreak response capabilities by expanding deployable RT-PCR capacity. Over the next few years this capacity will not need to be expanded. Instead, there will be a need for more centralized automated diagnostic capacity in order to increase throughput.

CAPACITY BUILDING

The AI supplemental funding has been used to strengthen NAMRU-3's internal capacity, which includes its service as the WHO Regional Influenza Reference Laboratory, and also its capacity in countries within the region, such as Jordan, Libya, Ghana, and Afghanistan, where NAMRU-3 has satellite laboratories (NAMRU-3, 2007b).

NAMRU-3 Laboratory Capacity

NAMRU-3 capacity has increased by adding additional BSL-3 space to fulfill a WHO terms-of-reference requirement to have one BSL-3 laboratory for animal-specimen processing and a separate facility for human specimens. NAMRU-3 has increased capacity for specimen processing by purchasing additional laboratory-based real-time PCR machines and adequate reagents and consumables to support any surge. NAMRU-3 has added technical staff to assist in both field and laboratory activities. In addition, four mobile RT-PCR machines were purchased to bolster outbreak-response capacity. NAMRU-3 is reportedly now capable of responding to four simultaneous outbreaks by providing forward laboratory support with appropriate personal protective equipment, reagents, and consumables for a sustained period.

Building Capacity of Regional Laboratory System and Training

NAMRU-3 has spent a significant amount of funding and effort on consulting with, training, and equipping more than 20 laboratories in the U.S. Central Command (CENTCOM) and U.S. European Command (EUCOM) areas of responsibility (see Figure 5.2). This was done in order to achieve the laboratories' capacity-building goal of creating a surveillance network that, with minimal continued support, can provide the necessary virological surveillance information for its own internal use while also contributing to the WHO-led global effort. To this end NAMRU-3 has expanded influenza surveillance expertise and diagnostic capacity throughout the region, including the countries of Azerbaijan, Djibouti, Egypt, Ghana, Iran, Iraq, Jordan, Kazakhstan, Kenya, Kyrgyzstan, Lebanon, Libya, Morocco, Nigeria, Oman, Pakistan, Saudi Arabia, Sudan, Syria, Ukraine, and Uzbekistan.

Capacity-building endeavors undertaken by NAMRU-3 generally incorporate a preliminary on-site assessment to determine the exact needs of the laboratory in terms of both infrastructure and expertise. NAMRU-3, WHO, FAO, various ministries of health, agriculture, and environment, DoD-GEIS headquarters, and other relevant partners determine how DoD-GEIS resources will be spent in the region. Capacity-building programs involving large-scale equipment placement take into account the geographic location of the laboratory, burden of disease, current political climate, location of deployed military forces, the location of NAMRU-3 assets, and other relevant factors. Capacity building involving training is prioritized and typically performed on a space-available basis. NAMRU-3 training will often be tailored to the laboratory capacity of the trainees' home country in such a way that NAMRU-3 can immediately put it to use. The timing of training is coordinated with the delivery of anticipated laboratory equipment via external grants (e.g., from the World Bank). NAMRU-3 also provides limited supplies and reagents, thereby facilitating immediate diagnostic capacity in the trainees' countries. Once NAMRU-3 has assisted in the establishment of the national influenza laboratories, oversight to ensure quality will continue at each of these locations as they further develop their skills.

NAMRU-3 has continued to work in this way with the Egyptian Ministries of Health and Environment to expand its surveillance and laboratory capacities.

In addition to its work in Egypt, NAMRU-3 has used the fiscal year 2006 DoD-GEIS-AI supplemental funding to substantially expand laboratory capacity in four targeted satellite laboratories in Jordan, Libya, Ghana, and Afghanistan. Equipment and reagents were purchased and delivered to all of these countries to establish their first national influenza centers. These sites, each of which has been assessed and will continue to receive equipment, supplies, and training as deemed appropriate by NAMRU-3 staff and national and global partners, will be capable of performing extensive diagnostics on both avian and seasonal influenza.

NAMRU-3 has delivered to Kabul, Afghanistan, all the necessary equipment (including four 6-foot biological safety cabinets) to set up two complete laboratories (one for the Ministry of Health and one for the Ministry of Agriculture). NAMRU-3 sent one medical repair technician to Kabul to oversee equipment installation and to certify the biological safety cabinets. After the equipment was in place, NAMRU-3 sent a molecular biologist to Kabul to conduct training in the laboratory itself. Currently there is a NAMRU-3 staff member temporarily assigned to Afghanistan.

Jordan has agreed to enter into the Trilateral Agreement with NAMRU-3 and the WHO. Under this agreement, NAMRU-3 is now training approximately three veterinarians a month from Jordan in avian influenza diagnostics.

After being requested to conduct an assessment of public health laboratory capacity in Libya, NAMRU-3 identified the laboratory site within the Center for Infectious Disease in Tripoli and oversaw the purchase of equipment and reagents. Equipment is slated to be trucked to Tripoli in the very near future. In addition there are plans for a medical repair technician to accompany the equipment in order to certify the biological safety cabinets prior to initiation of work. This certification is a biosafety initiative that NAMRU-3 imposed on all of the collaborating sites. In preparation for the opening of this laboratory site, NAMRU-3 hosted four Ph.D. scientists from Libya for a two-week hands-on training course on avian influenza diagnostics. This marked the first time NAMRU-3 has had Libyans training side-by-side with U.S. and Egyptian scientists.

Building on relationships established through NAMRU-3's detachment in Ghana, NAMRU-3 is supporting the establishment of a national influenza center in Accra, Ghana, located within the Noguchi Memorial Institute. All equipment and reagents have been purchased to outfit this site, and all of the previously used biological safety cabinets in its BSL-3 facility have been decontaminated and certified by NAMRU-3. All of the laboratory staff has been trained on-site in Ghana in molecular diagnostics as well as in viral isolation and typing.

In addition to the work undertaken at these four satellite labs, NAMRU-3 provides as-needed capacity building, training, and technical assistance to many other laboratories in the region. For example, NAMRU-3 conducted a brief collaboration with a laboratory site in Tbilisi, Georgia, which now functions almost independently. NAMRU-3 also scheduled a two-week influenza-related training for a Ph.D.-level Djibouti scientist, followed by additional on-site training in Djibouti City.

After the initial intensive assistance from NAMRU-3, countries should value and support their own laboratories. NAMRU-3 should transition to a technical assistance role—following up, providing quality assurance, and adding capacity as necessary through activities such as training.

Conclusions

NAMRU-3 has developed a process of assessing the needs of national laboratories, assisting in the acquisition of necessary equipment and supplies, training relevant laboratory staff, and providing follow-up technical assistance and confirmatory services as needed. This process has the potential to create sustainability and to establish a high-quality regional early warning system. WHO acts as a quality-control entity, and NAMRU-3 will have to continue to coordinate its activities with WHO and EMRO representatives. As NAMRU-3 establishes appropriate national laboratories in various countries in the EMRO region, it will need to move to a role more focused on follow up, confirmation of results, advanced virology, and quality assurance.

RECOMMENDATION 5-7. In order to assure the quality and sustainability of the regional influenza surveillance system, NAMRU-3 should work to establish standards and foundation documents for each of the steps in its laboratory-establishment process as well as to provide technical assistance for a new regional quality-assurance entity including (1) the development of a solid plan of strengthening regional countries' laboratory capacity with regard to avian influenza and maintaining this capacity through training, quality assurance, and proficiency testing; (2) continued collaboration with WHO to develop an external quality-assurance system for national central laboratories in the EMRO region; and (3) the use of NAMRU-3's extensive experience in capacity building (training, supervision, and mentoring) to develop structured (yet adaptable to each context) laboratory assessment checklists, training guidelines, and monitoring tools.

COLLABORATION AND COORDINATION

NAMRU-3 has many partners, including the Egyptian Ministries of Health, Environment, and Agriculture, governmental agencies of other countries in the EMRO region, other DoD departments, and a range of technical and financial partners such as the WHO and the CDC. NAMRU-3 is a WHO collaborating center for influenza. Information-sharing relationships between NAMRU-3 and its partners appear strong but seem to be informal, person-based, and circumstance-dependent.

Host Country Government

As a regional influenza reference laboratory, NAMRU-3 has the capacity to serve as a reference laboratory for all of the countries in the EMRO region, confirming influenza testing for ministries of health in the region. NAMRU-3 also extends assistance to the central Asian republics, West Africa, and countries such as Ukraine, Bulgaria, Macedonia, and Azerbaijan.

The Ministry of Health is the lead agent in Egypt's influenza surveillance effort. NAMRU-3 staff work very closely with representatives from the Ministry of Health, expanding the national human surveillance system and sharing results of laboratory testing on possible avian influenza samples. In addition, NAMRU-3 staff members participate at all coordination meetings with the Egyptian High Committee. The close relationship between NAMRU-3 and the Ministry of Health has enabled NAMRU-3 to work strategically and efficiently in Egypt in support of the national avian influenza surveillance network.

In terms of other Egyptian national partners, NAMRU-3 and the Egyptian Ministry of Environment have a strong collaborative relationship focused on the surveillance of migratory birds and routinely share information between each other, as NAMRU-3 performs all diagnostic assays.

While NAMRU-3 has collaborated with the Ministry of Agriculture on surge capacity for animal samples (specifically during outbreak situations) and for molecular characterization, their relationship needs strengthening. The Ministry of Agriculture shares limited information with relevant partners. This has made it difficult to bridge the gaps in information between human and wild bird surveillance activities being conducted by the Ministries of Health and Environment and supported by NAMRU-3.

In other countries where NAMRU-3 has ongoing influenza-related activities, it works directly with the ministries of health. These collaborations are based on mutual benefit. The national governments' commitment of personnel is instrumental in the timely collection and processing of influenza specimens. In turn, NAMRU-3's reporting of results significantly reduces response time. These relations typically result in positive outcomes both in terms of the expansion of influenza surveillance at the national and global levels and in terms of the medical diplomacy of the U.S. government in general.

Multilateral Agencies

Because of NAMRU-3's status as a WHO regional influenza reference laboratory, it works very closely with both EMRO and WHO headquarters in Geneva. This role was determined in collaboration with WHO and EMRO based on NAMRU-3's technical expertise and facilities capacity. NAMRU-3 is expected to become a WHO H5 reference center in the near future, which will strengthen even further its WHO regional and headquarters partnerships. At the current time, NAMRU-3 provides personnel and support to WHO and EMRO for outbreak investigations in the region. At WHO headquarters in Geneva, NAMRU-3 is a member of the Global Outbreak Alert Response Network (GOARN). NAMRU-3 staff routinely participate in the WHO regional pandemic/avian influenza meetings of EURO, EMRO, and AFRO (WHO Regional Office for Africa). They also conducted a WHO avian influenza training course for approximately 200 clinicians, laboratorians, and public health officials in Kiev for the countries of Ukraine, Azerbaijan, Georgia, Belarus, and Uzbekistan. No financial resources are regularly committed by WHO to NAMRU-3 as a WHO collaborating center. Currently, NAMRU-3 is using GEIS AI supplemental funding to perform all regional specimen processing, diagnostics, and characterization.

NAMRU-3 coordinates its animal-surveillance activities with FAO to ensure an optimal use of funds. FAO funding has been well complemented because it provided for a logistical base for field surveillance while the DoD-GEIS funding provided the resources to support reference laboratories, as in the case of the laboratory in Kabul.

U.S. Government Agencies

NAMRU-3 activities in Cairo, Egypt, are directly linked with the U.S. Department of State and other U.S. government agencies. Monthly reports and weekly updates are available to other U.S. government partners, such as CDC, HHS, and the U.S. Agency for International Development (USAID), and assist in coordinating efforts. As a WHO collaborating center, NAMRU-3 collaborates with the CDC and routinely sends the CDC avian influenza specimens for further characterization. The CDC has committed its time to processing and relaying information back to both NAMRU-3 and WHO-Geneva.

The upcoming assignment of CDC public health professionals to NAMRU-3 will strengthen its relationship with CDC as a key technical partner in Egypt. As of July 2007, NAMRU-3 was working with CDC to fill five positions at the laboratory including a senior epidemiologist to work as the director of the CDC International Emerging Infections Program (IEIP) in Cairo, an epidemiologist, a public health advisor, a Resident Advisor for the CDC Field Epidemiology Training Program, and a U.S. Public Health Service Captain to serve as influenza coordinator. NAMRU-3 staff expects that once the IEIP director is selected, administrative issues related to the organizational relationships will be determined collaboratively.

USAID is an additional collaborating partner of NAMRU-3 in a number of countries in which it conducts avian influenza activities. NAMRU-3 staff are routinely invited to USAID-sponsored meetings to provide input as regional experts. These meetings often lead to additional opportunities for avian influenza capacity building outside the regions in which NAMRU-3 is typically engaged. For Bulgaria and Macedonia, NAMRU-3 provided assistance with laboratory design, specimen-throughput consultation, and multiple training sessions, both at NAMRU-3 and in-country. Relations with USAID-Egypt seem to be less productive, though there are efforts under way to strengthen this collaboration.

Other DoD Entities

In terms of DoD in general, NAMRU-3's strategic location enables it to support CENTCOM, EUCOM, and a future AFCOM (U.S. African Command) with diagnostic support, outbreak response capacity, and training. To date, NAMRU-3 has been able to contribute by providing specimen collection to a number of military preventive medicine units in Iraq, Kuwait, Qatar, and Djibouti. In addition, NAMRU-3 has responded to outbreaks in Azerbaijan, Iraq, Sudan, and Djibouti.

Other DoD entities, such as the U.S. Army Medical Research Institute of Infectious Diseases (USAMRIID) and other military laboratories operating overseas, are also essential partners with NAMRU-3. There are a number of ongoing project-specific collaborations between NAMRU-3 and other DoD entities related to avian influenza. All reporting on regional efforts is sent to a variety of DoD offices in the United States, including DoD-GEIS headquarters, NMRC, and the Naval Bureau of Medicine and Surgery. NAMRU-3 also collaborates with USAMRIID by providing influenza RNA to assist USAMRIID in its development of future diagnostics. NAMRU-3 has worked extensively with the Naval Health Research Center to assist with specimen provision for the development of an electrospray ionization mass spectrometry device for respiratory pathogen identification. NAMRU-3 works with the Air Force Institute for Operational Health to provide accurate surveillance data. Using the supplemental funding, NAMRU-3 has also expanded its wild bird surveillance via their collaboration with DoD personnel at the U.S. Army Medical Research Unit-Kenya.

While there are certainly fruitful collaborations taking place between NAMRU-3 and other DoD entities, it was not completely clear to the IOM site visit team how communication and coordination with the DoD-GEIS headquarters and other DoD-GEIS sites is realized.

Private Organizations

The virology program at NAMRU-3 works with Idaho Technology Incorporated (ITI) to validate primer/probe sets dedicated for the military-deployable mobile real-time PCR systems. These will eventually be used to further support NAMRU-3's outbreak response. ITI provides limited supplies to conduct these validation studies, while DoD-GEIS AI supplemental funding covers labor costs and additional supplies. No cash resources are provided to NAMRU-3 by ITI.

Conclusions

NAMRU-3 has excellent long-term relationships with all of its partners in Egypt and the region. In particular, the AI/PI activities have increased the possibilities for capacity building with the Egyptian Ministry of Health in support of improved surveillance and response.

> **RECOMMENDATION 5-8. NAMRU-3 should continue to serve in a technical advisory role to the Egyptian Ministry of Health and carry out medical diplomacy by developing relationships with strategic partners while maintaining its role as an independent research agency with primary allegiances to the U.S. Navy.**

NAMRU-3 has been actively engaged in host country collaborations and is heavily committed in terms of personnel and resources in Egypt and the wider region. However, NAMRU-3 leadership stated that targets of opportunity often drive its activities, and this creates problems when trying to develop longer-range plans for the organization.

> **RECOMMENDATION 5-9. NAMRU-3 should develop country- and region-specific 3-year strategies that focus on host sustainability as well as on the development, expansion, and maintenance of an influenza early warning system.**

The committee encourages NAMRU-3 to continue its complementary and integrated relationship with CDC. The committee concluded that the development of a memorandum of understanding that defines roles and responsibilities and the chain of command would facilitate this relationship and related influenza activities at NAMRU-3. In addition, increased bilateral information sharing with USAID, including more collaboration on complementary activities such as development of information, education, and communication materials for AI awareness, could benefit the influenza activities of both U.S. agencies. These efforts to improve its collaboration with USAID could be facilitated by the U.S. mission.

REFERENCES

DoD-GEIS (Department of Defense Global Emerging Infections System). 2007a. *U.S. Naval Medical Research Unit No. 3.* http://www.geis.fhp.osd.mil/GEIS/Training/namru-3.asp (accessed June 12, 2007).

DoD-GEIS. 2007b. *Department of Defense influenza surveillance sites worldwide, 2007* (unpublished).

IOM (Institute of Medicine). 2001. *Perspectives on the Department of Defense Global Emerging Infections Surveillance and Response System: A program review.* Washington, DC: National Academy Press.

NAMRU-3. 2007a. *Estimated laboratory surge capacity* (unpublished).

NAMRU-3. 2007b. *Viral and zoonotic disease research program.* PowerPoint presentation presented during site visit March 4, 2007 Cairo, Egypt (unpublished).

NAMRU-3. 2007c. *Regional surveillance for influenza and other respiratory viruses in the Middle East, central Asia, Africa, and Eastern Europe.* PowerPoint presentation presented during site visit March 4, 2007 Cairo, Egypt (unpublished).

OIE (Organisation Mondiale de La Santé, World Organization for Animal Health). 2006. *Avian influenza in Egypt follow-up report No. 1.* http://www.oie.int/eng/info/hebdo/AIS_28.HTM#Sec7 (accessed June 12, 2007)

USDA (United States Department of Agriculture). 2006. *Avian influenza, Egypt: Impact Worksheet.* http://www.aphis.usda.gov/vs/ceah/cei/taf/iw_2006_files/foreign/hpaiegypt022306_files/hpaiegypt02232006bb.htm (accessed June 12, 2007).

WHO (World Health Organization). 2007a. *H5N1 avian influenza: Timeline of major events.* http://www.who.int/csr/disease/avian_influenza/Timeline_2007_03_20.pdf (accessed September 5, 2007).

WHO. 2007b. *Cumulative number of confirmed human cases of avian influenza A/(H5N1) reported to WHO.* http://www.who.int/csr/disease/avian_influenza/country/cases_table_2007_07_11/en/index.html (accessed September 5, 2007).

LIST OF CONTACTS

DoD-GEIS NAMRU-3 Assessment: Egypt

Adam Armstrong, Head Enteric Diseases Research Program, U.S. Naval Medical Research Unit No. 3

CAPT Bruce Boynton, Commanding Officer, U.S. Naval Medical Research Unit No. 3

David Hoel, Vector Biology research Program, U.S. Naval Medical Research Unit No. 3

Edward Kilbane, Head Disease Surveillance Research Program, U.S. Naval Medical Research Unit No. 3

Moustafa Mansour, Director of Research Sciences, U.S. Naval Medical Research Unit No. 3

Marshall Monteville, Head Viral and Zoonotic Diseases Research Program, U.S. Naval Medical Research Unit No. 3

Guillermo Pimentel, Disease Surveillance Research Program, U.S. Naval Medical Research Unit No. 3

Maha Talaat, Disease Surveillance Research Program, U.S. Naval Medical Research Unit No. 3

Jeff Tjaden, Viral and Zoonotic Diseases Research Program, U.S. Naval Medical Research Unit No. 3

Sam Yingst, Viral and Zoonotic Diseases Research Program, U.S. Naval Medical Research Unit No. 3

Matt Weiner, Enteric Diseases Research Program, U.S. Naval Medical Research Unit No. 3

Nasr EL-Sayed, First Under Secretary for Preventive and Endemic Affairs, Egyptian Ministry of Health and Population

Holly Fluty-Dempsey, Chief Population and Health Division, United States Agency for International Development

Akmal Elerian, Population and Health Division, United States Agency for International Development

Tara Milani, Population and Health Division, United States Agency for International Development

SCHEDULE OF EVENTS
DoD-GEIS NAMRU-3 Assessment

Cairo, Egypt
Participants: Mary J. R. Gilchrist
James Tibenderana
J. Alice Nixon
March 4-10, 2007

Sunday, March 4, 2007

0900-1000	**Greeting and command brief** Dr. Moustafa Mansour Lt. Stegall
1030-1030	**Tour of NAMRU-3** Dr. Moustafa Mansour
1130-1130	**Briefing on Enteric Diseases Research Program** Cdr. Adam Armstrong
1230-1230	Lunch
1400-1400	**Briefing on Disease Surveillance Program** Capt. Edward Kilbane
1600-1600	**Briefing on Viral and Zoonotic Diseases Research Program** Lt. Cdr. Marshall Monteville
1600-1630	Return to hotel

Monday, March 5, 2007

0700-0730	Depart NAMRU-3
0730-1430	**Visit to Damietta, Port Said, and Manzallah Lake field sites for migratory bird sampling**
1430-1700	Travel to Alexandria

Tuesday, March 6, 2007

1200-1200	**Visit to Alexandria Fever Hospital**
1400-1400	**Visit to field sites in Alexandria**
1730-1730	Return to Cairo

Wednesday, March 7, 2007

0900-1000	**Overview of field visits**
1000-1500	**Field visits to MoH, WHO (EMRO), USAID, DCM**
1500-	Return to hotel

Thursday, March 8, 2007

0830-0900	**Briefing with program heads**
0900-1000	**Overview of Vector Biology Research Program** Lt. Cdr. David Hoel
1000-1100	**Out-briefing and open discussion**
1600-	Return to hotel

Friday, March 9, 2007

0900-	**Optional tour**

Saturday, March 10, 2007

0900-	Departure

6

U.S. Army Medical Research Unit Kenya Avian and Pandemic Influenza Activities

In 1969 the U.S. Army Medical Research Unit Kenya (USAMRU-K), a special foreign activity of the Walter Reed Army Institute of Research in Washington, D.C., was activated on a temporary basis at the request of the government of Kenya to study trypanosomiasis (DoD-GEIS, 2007a). USAMRU-K's operations were originally dedicated to and supported by applied medical research, and its invitation to operate in Kenya was based on that research mission (IOM, 2001). Its operations became permanent in 1973, and since that time research has been conducted on malaria, leishmaniasis, and arboviruses (DoD-GEIS, 2007a). More recently, USAMRU-K has been involved with both avian and pandemic influenza surveillance (Schnabel, 2007).

Support for USAMRU-K influenza surveillance and response projects from the Department of Defense Global Emerging Infections Surveillance and Response System (DoD-GEIS) totaled approximately $3.5 million in fiscal year 2006 (2.6 million in AI/PI funds and $800 thousand in non-influenza DoD-GEIS funds) (USAMRU-K, 2007a). Using these funds, USAMRU-K built laboratory capacity at the Kenya Medical Research Institute (KEMRI) and other sites, established human surveillance projects in Kenya to detect influenza disease and gather much-needed information on the disease in sub-Saharan Africa, and began the processes of establishing similar influenza surveillance projects in Uganda and Cameroon[1] (Schnabel,

[1]At the time of the IOM team's visit the planning for the development of a DoD-GEIS influenza surveillance program in Cameroon was just beginning. For this reason no further details on this project are included in the chapter.

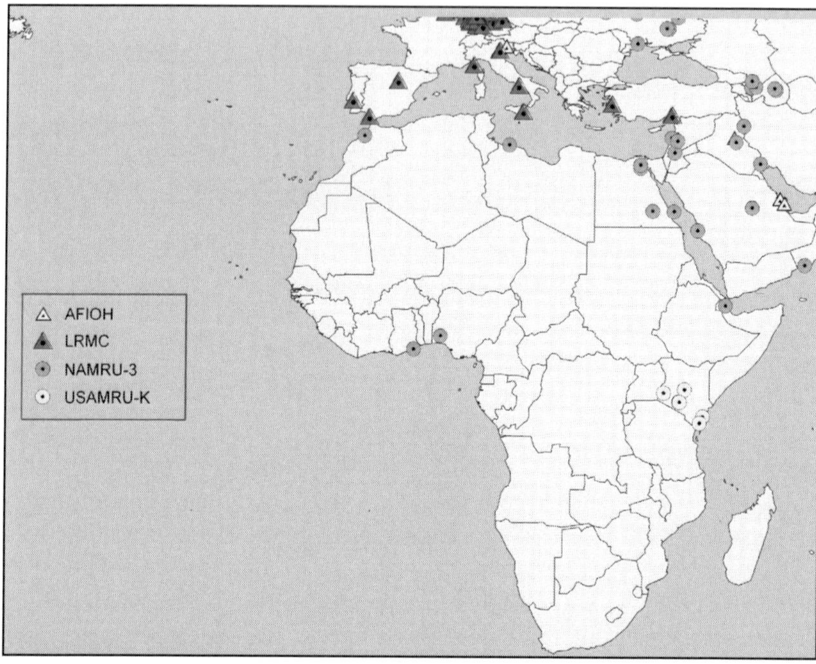

FIGURE 6-1 DoD's regional presence in influenza surveillance (Africa), 2007.
SOURCE: DoD-GEIS, 2007b.

2007) (see Figure 6-1). Migratory bird surveillance is also being conducted using DoD-GEIS avian influenza (AI) funds in conjunction with the Naval Medical Research Unit No. 3 (NAMRU-3) in Egypt.

A site visit team of the Institute of Medicine (IOM) Committee for the Assessment of DoD-GEIS Influenza Surveillance and Response Programs visited USAMRU-K from March 11-17, 2007.[2] A list of the people with whom the site visit team met and the itinerary that was followed can be found at the end of this chapter.

[2]Prior to the committee's visit to USAMRU-K, the laboratory staff provided the committee with detailed background information on USAMRU-K and the pandemic/avian influenza activities they were supporting. These materials are available from the IOM in the Public Access File.

INFLUENZA IN KENYA

Because of a lack of surveillance activities, little information is available about the disease characteristics of influenza in sub-Saharan Africa. At the time of the IOM visit, for example, it is unclear if there are seasonal outbreaks or what viruses are circulating in countries such as Kenya. Avian influenza has not yet been diagnosed in Kenya's wild birds or domestic poultry, but because of its situation and location the country has received considerable attention. Kenya lies along the migratory route of birds from Europe to southern Africa. In addition, it has water points that serve as stopovers for a variety of bird species. Kenya's poultry population is considerable—an estimated 30 million, 80 percent of which are indigenous backyard chickens (Kenya Red Cross Society, 2006).

Though there have been no outbreaks of avian influenza in the countries neighboring Kenya, both Nigeria and Egypt have reported human cases of avian influenza. In February 2006, Nigeria confirmed H5N1 in poultry, and a month later Niger, a country bordering Nigeria, also confirmed H5N1 in its domestic poultry. The first and so far only human case in Nigeria was confirmed in late January 2007. Egypt, having reported its first case of human influenza in March 2006, has since had a total of 35, the highest number of bird flu cases among humans outside of Asia (WHO, 2007a; WHO 2007b).

MANAGEMENT AND PLANNING

In developing avian influenza/pandemic influenza (AI/PI) projects, USAMRU-K staff drew on existing management tools. For example, preexisting mechanisms to manage the relationship between the staffs of USAMRU-K and the KEMRI lab, including a memorandum of understanding that covered laboratory staff's salaries, allowed USAMRU-K to quickly utilize AI/PI funding. USAMRU-K also signed a contract with the Henry M. Jackson Foundation, which included approximately $1.7 million of 2006 AI/PI funds, to develop and maintain influenza surveillance in Uganda and Cameroon and, potentially, other countries in the region. Current progress in developing the Uganda project is described in a separate section in this chapter.

Traditionally the DoD-GEIS coordinator was the principal investigator on all DoD-GEIS-related protocols. More recently, protocols have been amended to give primary scientific and management leadership to others, with the DoD-GEIS coordinator's position becoming more one of coordination and facilitation.

Using the supplemental funding, USAMRU-K has established a credible and highly professional biosafety level 2 (BSL-2) laboratory, which will be used for influenza surveillance activities well into the future. Once all planned surveillance sites are opened and the program is at full capacity, the Kenya flu program will require $800,000 per year, but this future expenditure has not been programmed into the USAMRU-K DoD-GEIS program outyear funding. Thus the DoD-GEIS core program at USAMRU-K would suffer drastic cuts if the supplementary flu program had to be absorbed into it.

Staffing

At the time of the IOM site visit team's visit, the USAMRU-K staff included nine Americans, a British immunologist, and a National Research Council Fellow, as well as two Kenyan physicians assigned temporarily from KEMRI. In addition there are usually several local and foreign graduate and postdoctoral students working there. The Kenyan technical staff numbers approximately 100. The commander of the Walter Reed Project (WRP) Kenya/USAMRU-K has 11 years experience in Kenya in 3 tours of duty. His relationships with the Ministry of Health (MoH) and KEMRI allow USAMRU-K to coordinate its work in Kenya and its interactions with the MoH and KEMRI seamlessly.

There were a number of dedicated members of USAMRU-K working on the DoD-GEIS AI/PI projects. Despite the DoD-GEIS coordinator's short time on the job (six months), the IOM site visit team was impressed with his grasp of the DoD-GEIS programmatic situation in Kenya. The virologist responsible for day-to-day DoD-GEIS influenza laboratory activities had considerable postdoctoral experience in animal virology in the United Kingdom prior to his return to Kenya. The WRP veterinarian who oversees surveillance for influenza virus in wild birds works closely with collaborators at NAMRU-3.

Overall the USAMRU-K staff has administered the AI/PI program well. USAMRU-K would greatly benefit from additional administrative help for DOD-GEIS protocols. Because the AI/PI funds are so constrained with respect to when they arrive, how they are to be used, and the limited time in which they must be committed, an important function of the administrator would be to help USAMRU-K project officers allocate AI/PI funding more efficiently to appropriate activities within the allotted calendar interval.

Many of USAMRU-K's AI/PI projects have Kenyan principal investigators. Furthermore, all of the project and laboratory staff are Kenyan, ensuring that Kenya will retain the technical capacity to continue the surveillance in the future. In addition, the USAMRU-K staff working in the National Influenza Center (NIC) on influenza surveillance receive the same salaries as their counterparts being paid by KEMRI. This parity in salaries ensures that KEMRI can afford to take up the salaries of these staff if control of the laboratory is turned over to Kenya.

Technology and Information Management

Technology and information management for the USAMRU-K/DoD-GEIS influenza project are in their formative stages. The specimen recording is currently done all by hand. Fortunately, the influenza program can draw on existing expertise in this area from other WRP/DoD-GEIS protocols to improve its data management and to fast track the necessary improvements. In addition, there are plans for the WRP to obtain a $30,000 sophisticated freezer-management software and bar-coding system, which will help manage the storage and tracking of influenza (as well as all other) specimens.

Conclusions

The supplemental AI/PI funding received in fiscal year 2006 was successfully utilized to establish functional influenza surveillance despite a significant delay in receiving the funds. This success demonstrates the flexibility and robustness of the administrative infrastructure at USAMRU-K. To maximize AI/PI funds, USAMRU-K would benefit from an additional administrator to help manage the finances of the AI/PI projects.

The current USAMRU-K staff appears to be adequate for the current influenza protocols but may be inadequate if the program is to expand. To do longer-term surveillance USAMRU-K would need a mechanism to pay people for longer periods. The annual funding cycles challenge USAMRU-K staff in their ability to plan protocols and staffing beyond one to two years. This challenge of middle-term planning is exacerbated by the short tours of the Army leadership, which often limit Army personnel to tours of two to three years.

The basic technological capabilities at USAMRU-K are sufficient, but there is a great need to expand the information systems for sample handling. USAMRU-K has already identified this as a need and is currently researching various options. The IOM site visit team considered the investment in a specimen cataloguing and tracking system to be a wise use of DoD-GEIS money as it will benefit all of WRP's activities, improving the handling of specimens generated there as well as those from DoD-GEIS influenza surveillance.

SURVEILLANCE

In Kenya, there are ongoing (or soon-to-commence) surveillance activities supported by DoD-GEIS supplemental funding to detect influenza disease, to perform virologic confirmation, and to isolate influenza viruses in wild bird populations and in human populations.

Human Surveillance

The DoD-GEIS influenza surveillance in Kenya aims to isolate and characterize influenza viruses circulating among human populations, to estimate the burden of influenza disease among Kenyan children and adults, and to identify other viral and bacterial agents causing acute respiratory illnesses (USAMRU-K, 2007c). The DoD-GEIS-supported national surveillance system complements influenza surveillance activities being carried out by the Emerging Infections Program of the Centers for Disease Prevention and Control (CDC) in conjunction with KEMRI. CDC surveillance is aimed at detecting more severe clinical forms of influenza among hospitalized patients, while the WRP surveillance is directed at detecting influenza among less severely ill ambulatory patients seen as outpatients.

At the time of the IOM site visit, the surveillance protocol was designed to collect specimens from a maximum of five patients a day ranging in age from 2 months to adult who present at one of five designated outpatient facilities with fever of at least 38°C plus sore throat or cough, and with the onset of illness having occurred within the previous 72 hours (Bulimo, 2007). A questionnaire is administered to collect demographic information along with data on whether other household members have had respiratory illness, if the patient has recently traveled, and if the patient has a history of contact with chickens or other birds. Informed consent is obtained before collecting the demographic and clinical data and the specimens. Two duplicate nasopharyngeal swabs are obtained and put into a transport medium and cultured on Madin-Darby canine kidney (MDCK) cells. From July 2006 through February 2007, a total of 806 specimens were collected. Presently, DoD-GEIS surveillance sites are located throughout the country, clustered according to population densities, and the number of surveillance sites is planned to be expanded (USAMRU-K, 2007c).

Since little is known about the seasonality of influenza in tropical populations or about the importance of influenza as a cause of acute respiratory disease in relation to other viral and bacterial respiratory agents in children and adults, epidemiologists at the Kenyan MoH have been urging DoD-GEIS investigators to use the influenza surveillance as an opportunity to investigate in the same patients the co-occurrence of other viral and bacterial pathogens hours (Bulimo, 2007). Given the keen interest of the MoH in obtaining such etiologic data, the IOM team was supportive of nesting a study to detect an array of other viral and bacterial etiologies within the influenza surveillance activities. Should such a modification to the protocol proceed, it would be advisable to also collect respiratory specimens from age-matched healthy controls without acute respiratory illness, as a number of known respiratory pathogens can be present in non-ill individuals who have subclinical infection. Quantifying the background of such subclinical infection for various pathogens would be invaluable in allowing the most comprehensive analysis and interpretation of the surveillance data for influenza as well as for other etiologies.

Conclusions

Overall, the IOM Committee found that USAMRU-K's human surveillance projects in Kenya were well planned and executed. However, the site visit team suggested several areas in which the designs of the projects could be improved. One suggestion was to collect two sets of specimens each day at each site: one set of five specimens from children less than 60 months of age and the other set from children older than 60 months and adults. The significance of this is that acute respiratory illness from a variety of different respiratory agents is common in young children. Thus, for example, a circulating respiratory syncytial virus (RSV) epidemic occurring at the same time as circulation of influenza viruses could mask detection of the latter if mostly young children were sampled to the exclusion of older children and adults. Having independent collections of specimens from young children as well as from older children and adults would make such problems less likely. In these young pediatric patients the site visit team also suggested using reverse transcription polymerase chain reaction (RT-PCR) to test stool specimens from patients with gastroenteritis in order to detect H5 influenza virus.

Several of the current surveillance sites provide opportunities to test specimens from pediatric and adult patients with acute respiratory illness for other viruses (e.g., RSV A and B, parainfluenza viruses 1, 2, and 3, adenovirus, and human metapneumovirus) and bacterial pathogens (e.g., *Haemophilus influenzae* type b, *Streptococcus pneumoniae*—which should be serotyped—and *Bordetella pertussis*) in addition to H5, H3, H1, B, and other influenza viruses. If a broader search for etiologic agents is undertaken, the study should also include collection of specimens from age-matched healthy controls. Such data would elucidate the relative importance of influenza viruses at different times of the year in different age groups in comparison with other pathogens. Having data from controls would also allow an estimate of the relative pathogenicity of the different agents by comparing detection of agents in cases versus controls.

Because of an outbreak of influenza detected in western Kenya that caused the closure of schools due to a high absentee rate, the team suggested that a surveillance system be established in schools located near the current clinical surveillance sites in order to monitor absenteeism. If cooperation from the local school headmasters, headmistresses, and teachers can be obtained, a threshold of absenteeism could be set. If the threshold is surpassed, this would be an indication for a small team from the nearby clinical facility to visit schools and collect upper respiratory specimens from ill children (at school and at their homes). This form of surveillance would also build capacity in conducting outbreak investigation and in the collection of specimens during outbreaks. Beyond the improvements to existing surveillance activities, USAMRU-K should explore linkages with school surveillance and expansion into respiratory surveillance in the Kenyan military population.

Kenyan military populations have many young adults housed under crowded conditions, so that stringent surveillance for respiratory infections can usually be maintained. In the United States, there have been multiple instances where the onset of epidemic influenza was first detected (and the virus type identified) through detection of outbreaks among military personnel on installations or in military academies.

RECOMMENDATION 6-1. The total number of adults and children each day who present to the clinics with acute respiratory illness for specimen collection under the current protocol should be logged, even though only five young children and five older children or adults will be sampled. By recording the total number of such patients and having the proportion of the five-patient samples that are positive, an estimate can be made of the burden of disease leading persons to seek attention at the sentinel health care facilities. Without collecting the number of syndromic eligible cases, burden cannot be estimated.

RECOMMENDATION 6-2. To foster collaboration and illustrate the value of the surveillance activities to stakeholders, USAMRU-K should consider supporting a weekly or biweekly summary of the number of cases of acute respiratory illness and of influenza virus isolations, by age group, to be sent to all the surveillance sites to provide feedback to the clinicians involved in the surveillance system.

Animal Surveillance

Kenya contains part of three flyways for birds migrating from Europe and Asia (Limbaso, 2007). The routes are the western flyway (west of the Rift Valley), the eastern flyway (east of the Rift Valley), and the Rift Valley flyway. In Egypt, scientists at NAMRU-3 were trapping migrating birds and collecting cloacal swabs to detect influenza viruses. The NAMRU-3 scientists contacted Walter Reed and Kenyan scientists to elicit their interest in collaborating to extend that surveillance to the flyways in Kenya. A collaborative protocol was prepared by a local Kenyan principal investigator. A specific focus of the surveillance project, conceived in early 2004 and initiated in October 2005, is to detect highly pathogenic H5 and H7 (or other highly pathogenic) influenza viruses. The main ornithine targets of this surveillance are ducks and other waders as they migrate from Europe and Asia. It is anticipated that this surveillance can identify sites and situations where spillover can occur to local bird populations (including domestic chickens) and to human populations (Limbaso, 2007). The epidemiologic concern is that migratory birds carrying highly pathogenic influenza viruses can transmit the avian viruses to domestic waterfowl or domestic chickens. Infections in domestic chickens could, in turn, lead to cross-species infection of humans.

Migratory bird study sites were selected based on the frequency of the targets (wild ducks and waders). The migration season typically extends from October through March. The 10 sites sampled include (Limbaso, 2007)

- sewage ponds in Nairobi, Nakuru (near Lake Nakuru in the Rift Valley, northwest of Nairobi, halfway to Lake Victoria), and Thika (Central Kenya, about 100 kilometers north of Nairobi);
- lakes along the Rift Valley;
- swamps around Nairobi; and
- dams in the central highlands.

Birds are trapped and handled by qualified ornithologists; the traps used include wader mist nets, modified Balchiari traps, and door traps. Birds are ringed and classified by species, and various biometric measurements are made. Duplicate cloacal samples are collected by the DoD-GEIS veterinarian, preserved in transport medium in liquid nitrogen (-80°C), and transported to the laboratory for virologic processing. All samples are screened for influenza A viruses by RT-PCR in the BSL-3 laboratory on the KEMRI campus, maintained by the CDC Emerging Infections Program in conjunction with KEMRI (Limbaso, 2007). Any H5 isolates are forwarded to NAMRU-3 in Cairo for further characterization. At NAMRU-3 the RT-PCR is confirmed, and, once confirmation is obtained, the samples are cultured in eggs. Subtyping is carried out using kits supplied by the CDC influenza branch.

During the last migration season, 438 birds representing 38 different species were sampled. Of these specimens, 24 (5.5 percent) yielded influenza A viruses, including one H5N3 isolate of low pathogenicity (Limbaso,

2007). The IOM site visit team discussed with the WRP veterinarian the possibility of performing tracheal cultures as well as cloacal cultures on the larger species of birds. The USAMRU-K-supported team did not have experience with tracheal cultures of birds and was somewhat hesitant to perform these because of concerns that they might inadvertently injure the birds. Accordingly, the IOM site visit team mentioned to the Kenyan scientists that NAMRU-2 scientists in Indonesia were carrying out a similar surveillance of wild birds in which tracheal cultures and blood from a wing vein were being obtained in addition to cloacal cultures. The IOM site visit team discussed with WRP Kenya staff the possibility of visiting NAMRU-2 to learn how scientists there perform tracheal cultures.

At the present time, there is no systematic surveillance for influenza viruses among either domestic chickens or industrial poultry farm chickens in Kenya. However, there is the intent and capability to perform outbreak investigations, including collection of specimens for diagnostic tests, should there occur a die-off of chickens, either among backyard poultry or industrial farm birds.

Conclusions

While animal influenza surveillance conducted by USAMRU-K in conjunction with NAMRU-3 represents a solid start, the committee concluded that USAMRU-K would benefit from additional guidance from other DoD OCONUS (outside the continental United States) laboratories in order to increase the value of the activities currently being performed and to expand the relative expertise of the USAMRU-K staff on the ground.

RECOMMENDATION 6-3. USAMRU-K should draw on the experience of other DoD OCONUS laboratories in animal influenza surveillance. For example, the USAMRU-K veterinarian could be sent to NAMRU-2 in Indonesia to gain experience in performing tracheal cultures on trapped wild birds.

LABORATORY

Influenza surveillance in Kenya is a collaborative effort between USAMRU-K, KEMRI, the Kenyan MoH, CDC's International Emerging Infectious Disease Program-Kenya, and the World Health Organization (WHO). The WHO-designated National Influenza Center (NIC) laboratory is located on the KEMRI campus in Nairobi and is operated jointly by USAMRU-K and KEMRI. Each of the collaborators has a very clearly defined role so as to avoid overlapping and duplicating activities. USAMRU-K provides the laboratory director and support for eight technical staff, while KEMRI provides the facilities and two additional technicians. CDC provides two technicians for operation of real-time PCR. Both the KEMRI and CDC staff may be pulled out of the laboratory for emergencies, such as the recent Rift Valley Fever outbreak. USAMRU-K conducts outpatient influenza virus surveillance at five sites. CDC operates the BSL-3 laboratory in the KEMRI facility and conducts hospital-based surveillance at five sites. All respiratory samples collected in both the CDC and USAMRU-K surveillance programs are received and processed by the NIC. The MoH is the regulatory authority and ultimate recipient of the data generated by NIC.

The IOM site visit team was unable to visit the laboratory in Nairobi because of a temporary security-related travel restriction at the time of the visit but was informed that the existing NIC facilities had been completely stripped and refurbished and new equipment installed. The laboratory resumed operation in 2006, and testing of surveillance samples began in July 2006. The anticipated workload is approximately 200 samples per week, which is a large volume for a complete tissue culture workup on all samples.

The laboratory operates under BSL-2 conditions with two Class 2 biosafety cabinets. Laboratory diagnosis is currently performed using tissue culture systems with isolates identified by conventional serologic techniques. Diagnostic capabilities exist for influenza viruses, adenoviruses, enteroviruses, parainfluenza viruses, human metapneumovirus, and RSV. Real-time PCR is expected to be fully operational in the NIC before the end of March. Thus it is expected that by April 2007 all samples collected under the outpatient surveillance program supported by USAMRU-K, as well as samples collected under the inpatient program supported by CDC, will be screened by RT-PCR for influenza A and B and H5 using specific primers. Samples positive for A or B from the outpatient project will be further serotyped from cultures. Influenza-positive samples from the inpatient study will be forwarded to CDC for further workup. Any sample positive for H5 from any human source will be immediately forwarded to the BSL-3 facility without further NIC workup.

Influenza viruses isolated to date by the NIC have been sent with original samples to the Air Force Institute for Operational Health (AFIOH) facility in San Antonio for confirmation and virus sequencing. However, shipments to the United States are reportedly expensive (approximately $2,000). Sending isolates to NAMRU-3 was proposed as an alternative.

NIC provides weekly and monthly reports to USAMRU-K and to KEMRI, which in turn reports to the MoH. This reporting mechanism is organizationally appropriate but may lead to delays in relaying information. A mechanism for real-time feedback to the site-collaborating physicians has yet to be decided upon. Relationships with KEMRI are good, but the reporting process leaves little opportunity for the NIC to interact with the MoH.

The reporting channels to WHO were unclear to the IOM site visit team. The designation of the laboratory as a National Influenza Center carries with it the obligation to participate fully in the global influenza network. This means the national government is expected to promptly report isolation of influenza viruses to WHO and promptly forward representative isolates to WHO-designated reference laboratories.

NIC is not directly involved in the NAMRU-3 wild bird surveillance project. All specimens are submitted directly to the CDC/KEMRI BSL-3 facility for further workup. Samples collected by veterinarians from suspected poultry outbreaks, from sick or dead birds, or from other MoH wild bird surveys are submitted to the Veterinary Institute Laboratory in Kabete, Kenya. The team was informed that Kabete has RT-PCR capability, with equipment and training provided by CDC.

Conclusions

Even though the site visit team did not get a chance to tour the USAMRU-K laboratory facilities in Nairobi, based on the description of the laboratory the site visit team felt that USAMRU-K was making good progress in the establishment and improvement of the National Influenza Center operating in collaboration with KEMRI. The NIC is in a unique position to contribute to the knowledge of specific viral and bacterial agents in respiratory disease in the children of Kenya. Multiplex PCR and RT-PCR methodologies offer the possibility of performing such studies in a systematic way by testing samples at selected surveillance sites using an automated PCR-based machine. Advantages of such an approach include simplification of quality control, a high level of automation, and the ability to detect a broad array of etiologic agents. Downsides include the high cost of initial capital investment for such a machine, high operating costs, and questions about the sustainability of operating such a machine should KEMRI have to take on this responsibility in the future.

RECOMMENDATION 6-4. USAMRU-K should consider the expansion of laboratory capacity to include multitasking diagnostic equipment for respiratory diseases.

RESPONSE CAPACITY

Surge Capacity

With the arrival in April of the real-time RT-PCR machine, the National Influenza Center at KEMRI operated by USAMRU-K will shortly be capable of carrying out molecular screening on 200 samples per week (see

TABLE 6-1 Summary of Surge Capability at USAMRU-K

Condition	NIC Lab	VHF lab	Kondele Research Lab	Total Samples
Routine operation	200/week	0/week	0/week	200/week
Altered algorithm (Flu A & H5 first)	1,000/week	500/week	500/week	2,000/week
Target H5 gene only	1,000/week	500/week	500/week	2,000/week
24-hours–a-day, seven-days-a-week operations	2,000/week	1,000/week	1,000/week	4,000/week

SOURCE: USAMRU-K, 2007b.

Table 6-1). Field sites only have rudimentary laboratory capabilities and are not able to screen additional samples (USAMRU-K, 2007b).

In a periepidemic situation, the initial NIC response would be to change the current algorithm to test for influenza A and H5. With the use of the multiplexing capability of the RT- PCR machine, USAMRU-K would then be able to screen for an additional 800 samples per week at the NIC. Furthermore, in the case of an epidemic, two additional labs within the USAMRU-K DoD-GEIS program would be recruited to augment flu screening: the WHO Regional Reference Laboratory for Arbovirology and Viral Hemorrhagic Fever (KEMRI main campus in Nairobi), which is already a primary DoD-GEIS program laboratory, and the USAMRU-K Kondele research laboratory, which was toured by the IOM site visit team. These two labs could each process an additional 500 samples per week, bringing the total capacity to 2,000 samples per week in a periepidemic situation. Obviously this would require reassigning staff from other programs in viral hemorrhagic fever (VHF) and Kondele research labs to process flu samples (USAMRU-K, 2007b).

Further refinement of the screening process to target only the gene required to rule in or rule out the subtype would not alter the numbers of samples screened per week because USAMRU-K assumed the utilization of the multiplex capacity above.

If required, USAMRU-K could operate 24 hours a day, seven days a week, doubling its capacity at all three laboratories. This would bring the total number of samples processed by USAMRU-K to 4,000 per week. Again, this would require reassigning staff from other programs in VHF and Kondele research labs to maintain the 24-hours-a-day, seven-days-a-week operations and would require equipment to be on standby in case of a primary equipment failure. USAMRU-K does not currently stock reagents to process such high samples loads. A stockpile of reagents and laboratory consumables has been budgeted using fiscal year 2007 funds (USAMRU-K, 2007b).

In the event of a large-scale epidemic, CDC-Kenya would probably take the U.S. government agencies' lead. CDC's laboratory and supply capability would probably double surge capacity in Kenya. The Wellcome Trust laboratory would also probably participate in outbreak response on the coast.

The National Plan of Action for Preparedness and Response to Avian Influenza in Uganda (April 2006) describes the steps necessary to achieve national response readiness. Uganda participated with Kenya in the combined WHO/Food and Agricultural Organization (FAO)/CDC training-of-trainers program, but the country lacks the necessary resources to continue in-country training at the same rate as Kenya. Spokespersons for the MoH estimated that the goals of the national plan are roughly 10 percent complete. The national plan is currently under review to document progress, identify major program gaps, revise funding needs, and assign priorities for implementation. The major challenges are still the limited financial and human resources (USAMRU-K, 2007b).

Conclusions

While there have not been any cases of avian influenza in Kenya, USAMRU-K has a history of participating in infectious disease outbreak investigations alongside the MoH and CDC representatives and has a well developed surge capacity plan in the event that an avian outbreak does occur.

CAPACITY BUILDING

In fiscal year 2006, the supplemental funding was used to strengthen the NIC's BSL-2 laboratory at KEMRI, including the purchase of a PCR machine (Bulimo, 2007).

In addition to the development of the NIC laboratory, USAMRU-K conducted an influenza training course held May 3-11, 2006, at the Walter Reed DoD-GEIS laboratories at KEMRI. This was the first training course conducted by the flu program, and classes covered basic science and practical topics. The USAMRU-K flu staff attended as well as representatives from Cameroon, Uganda, Burundi, and Kenya. In total, 21 participants were given training that consisted of two components, a theoretical element and a practical element. The theoretical aspect included the historical context of influenza, the epidemiology of influenza, good laboratory practice, laboratory safety, personal protective equipment, specimen collection and handling, polymerase chain reactions as a diagnostic tool for influenza, and outbreak management. The practical aspect covered cell culture practicum, specimen collection practicum, inoculation of virus samples (including known positives) into MDCK cells, identification of cytopathic effect (CPE) in influenza virus-infected cells, harvest of influenza viruses from infected cell cultures, cryopreservation of MDCK cells as well as virus isolates, and hemagglutinin/human avian influenza practicum.

A field trip to a bird breeding and feeding location at the Ruai sewage plant in Nairobi was organized in conjunction with personnel from the National Museums of Kenya to trap birds and collect cloacal swabs. A sacred ibis caught by this team at the Jomo Kenyatta International Airport was brought to KEMRI. All procedures ranging from tagging of the bird to biometric measurements and the collection of cloacal swabs were demonstrated by the veterinarian attached to USAMRU-K together with staff from the National Museums of Kenya. At the end of the training course, certificates of participation were presented to all involved.

The training course participants were selected because they plan to have direct involvement with USAMRU-K influenza surveillance programs. In addition, the training course incorporated pretests and posttests to evaluate the participants' comprehension of the course. The participants who work within the USAMRU-K flu program have demonstrated understanding and knowledge of influenza, but otherwise there has been no mechanism to evaluate how beneficial the training has been.

Conclusions

In collaboration with KERMI and CDC, USAMRU-K has increased the laboratory capacity of the Kenyan NIC by training staff, strengthening BSL-2 performance, and adding PCR capabilities. USAMRU-K has contributed to building laboratory capacity elsewhere in sub-Saharan Africa by participating in training laboratory technicians from a variety of countries.

COLLABORATION AND COORDINATION

Influenza surveillance in Kenya is a collaborative effort between USAMRU-K (DoD), KEMRI, the Kenyan MoH, CDC's International Emerging Infections Program-Kenya (IEIP), and WHO. USAMRU-K also participates on the Kenyan influenza taskforce with the Ministry of Livestock and Fisheries, represented by the Central Investigation Laboratories; the Ministry of Health, represented by the Director of Medical Services; research institutes and bodies (KEMRI, USAMRU-K, CDC-Kenya); the ornithology department of the National Museums of Kenya; the Kenya Wildlife Service; and funding bodies such as WHO, the U.S. Agency for

International Development, the German Agency for Technical Cooperation, and the FAO. Committees have been formed within this task force, and each is responsible for different aspects such as surveillance, prevention, laboratory support, infection control, and control and eradication.

Collaborative operation of the WHO-designated NIC laboratory allows for extremely close coordination between USAMRU-K and KEMRI. To facilitate information sharing, the NIC provides weekly and monthly reports to USAMRU-K and to KEMRI, which is responsible for reporting to the MoH. This reporting mechanism is organizationally appropriate but may lead to delays in relaying information. A mechanism for real-time feedback to the site-collaborating physicians has yet to be decided upon. Relationships with KEMRI are good, but the reporting process leaves little opportunity for the NIC to interact with the MoH.

USAMRU-K collaborates with CDC-IEIP in Kenya, with Kenya's MoH and Ministry of Livestock and Fisheries, and with NAMRU-3 in Cairo in conducting a migratory bird surveillance program.

In addition to current collaborations, USAMRU-K is exploring the development of an influenza-related protocol with the Kenya Department of Defense.

The designation of the laboratory as a National Influenza Center carries with it the obligation to participate fully in the global influenza network on a timely basis. This means the national government is expected to promptly report isolation of influenza viruses to WHO and promptly forward representative isolates to WHO-designated reference laboratories.

Conclusions

USAMRU-K is working closely with relevant partners in Kenya to implement avian influenza activities. These relationships have benefited both USAMRU-K and the host country.

However, the site visit team was unclear about the sharing of USAMRU-K findings and isolates with the global influenza information network and the communication channels to any WHO entity in terms of planned expansion of the African influenza surveillance network. This becomes a larger concern as USAMRU-K expands into other countries in the region.

RECOMMENDATION 6-5. Based on the close proximity of laboratory space at KEMRI and the potential overlap in influenza activities, USAMRU-K should increase its efforts to facilitate communications between principal investigators at the USAMRU-K/NIC and CDC and the staff of the two laboratories, including joint seminars, data sharing, and cross training on equipment and BSL-3 principles and practices. As part of this communication, USAMRU-K and the NIC should develop

a written understanding among all partners concerning WHO expectations about the reporting of influenza virus isolations and appropriate communication channels.

The site visit team saw a number of examples of close collaborations between USAMRU-K and CDC during the site visit. However, there seemed also to be a number of disconnects between the two U.S. entities, which may represent lost opportunities for efficiency.

UGANDA

The proposed Uganda program would involve surveillance for H5 and other influenza viruses, including obtaining cloacal cultures from captured migrating waterfowl and assaying for influenza viruses; epidemiological and virologic investigation of chicken die-offs; and detection of influenza virus infections among a systematic sample of pediatric and adult ambulatory patients who present with acute respiratory illnesses to the outpatient department of Mulago Hospital in Kampala or to rural Kayunga District Hospital (Wabwire-Mangen, 2007). The proposed USAMRU-K project in Uganda is to be administered through the Makerere University Walter Reed Project (MUWRP). Several Walter Reed Project staff members are on the ground facilitating the planning and coordination with Ugandan government officials (Wabwire-Mangen, 2007).

Proposed Human Influenza Surveillance Project in Uganda

A professor from Makerere University is the nominated principal investigator of the proposed DoD-GEIS-supported human influenza surveillance project. The surveillance plan is to enroll eligible pediatric subjects (age 2 months to 12 years) and adult subjects at two health care facilities, the urban Mulago National Referral and Teaching Hospital in Kampala and the rural Kayunga District Hospital. At Mulago the plan is to seek out pediatric patients with acute respiratory illness from among ambulatory patients seeking health care at the assessment center (i.e., the triage facility in the outpatient department) or at the pediatric acute care unit, an adjacent unit where more seriously ill children who are not directly admitted to the hospital can stay under clinical observation for up to 24 hours (after which they are either admitted to the inpatient pediatric service or discharged to home) (Wabwire-Mangen, 2007). Similarly, adult outpatients with more severe acute respiratory illness are diverted from the triage area of the outpatient department and kept under observation in the accident and emergency unit. After a period of observation, the adult patients are either admitted to the hospital or discharged to home. At Kayunga Hospital specimens will be obtained from eligible pediatric and adult patients with acute respiratory illness seen either in the outpatient department or admitted to the hospital (Wabwire-Mangen, 2007).

Eligible patients include children (age 2 months to 12 years) and adults who present with fever greater than 38°C, oral or axillary, with cough or sore throat, and with an onset of illness within the previous 72 hours (Wabwire-Mangen, 2007). The IOM site visit team was informed that the protocol intended to exclude pregnant women and patients with exudative tonsillitis or pharyngitis. The IOM team was told that a total of up to five specimens per day would be obtained from patients both at Mulago and at Kayunga.

As part of the surveillance protocol, demographic data, clinical information, and a history of travel or animal contact (particularly with chickens) will be collected from each patient. Clinical specimens will be processed in the refurbished microbiology laboratory of the Veterinary School of Makerere University to detect the presence of influenza viruses. Data entry will be performed at MUWRP.

Migrating Waterfowl Surveillance in Uganda

Nature Uganda, a nongovernmental agency that is the local affiliate of Bird International, has been monitoring the numbers and species of migrating waterfowl that land in various regions of Uganda including (1) the western Rift Valley lakes (Queen Elizabeth Conservation Area, Kyambura Wildlife Reserve, Murchison Falls National Park); (2) the Lake Victoria region (eastern, central, and southwestern shorelines, Lake Mburo, and Sango Bay): and (3) the eastern Uganda wetlands (Lake Kyoga, Lake Opeta, Lake Bisina, and two Uganda rice schemes, Kibimda and Doho) (Wabwire-Mangen, 2007). At these sites Nature Uganda workers have found migrating waterfowl in close proximity to indigenous birds, including ducks.

USAMRU-K intends to partner with Nature Uganda and to expand the activities to include the collection of cloacal swabs. These swabs will be tested for influenza viruses including H5N1. Any influenza virus isolates will be sent to the WHO International Influenza Virus Reference Laboratory for viruses of animal origin (Wabwire-Mangen, 2007).

Although USAMRU-K does not currently have plans to conduct surveillance on domestic birds, the government of Uganda does have a protocol in place for die-offs. If information reaches the Ministry of Agriculture of a die-off of chickens or of other birds, an investigative team will be sent to obtain specimens and gather information. The specimens will be tested to determine if highly pathogenic influenza viruses are responsible for the severe and fatal disease.

Proposed USAMRU-K Laboratory in Uganda

The IOM team visited one of the potential sites under consideration by USAMRU-K for assisting Uganda in developing laboratory surveillance capacity. The site is located on the campus of Makerere University in the School of Veterinary Medicine. Proposed space in the 30-year-old building is poorly designed and ill equipped, but it could be adequately renovated to meet requirements for a BSL-2 laboratory. Laboratory staff would need to be hired and trained; no virology professionals are currently associated with the laboratory. Achieving a fully functioning laboratory to support the proposed human and avian surveillance studies will require considerable investment.

Uganda officials fully support the expansion of influenza surveillance capabilities as proposed by USAMRU-K and agree in principle on the proposed surveillance protocol and possible sites for sample collection. Details of the laboratory arrangement remain to be resolved. Resolution depends, in part, on an extended visit to the Uganda Virus Research Institute (UVRI) to assess its current activities and capabilities, national and global obligations, interest in expanding influenza virus surveillance, and possible role in the proposed USAMRU-K project.

Currently, the Ministry of Agriculture, Animal Industry, and Fisheries (MAAIF) is assigned responsibility, in collaboration with the Ugandan Wildlife Authority, for surveillance, situation monitoring, and assessment activities in animals. (The MoH is assigned responsibility for establishing and implementing systems for prevention and containment of influenza in humans.) MAAIF currently monitors the occurrence of important disease threats in wild and domestic animal populations, but it will require considerable strengthening in order to meet its responsibilities for AI. MAAIF has no avian influenza diagnostic capabilities itself and in the case of avian influenza relies on the UVRI, which is designated the WHO National Influenza Center. The UVRI is responsible for rapid analysis and sharing of specimens or isolates for (influenza) virus characterization and development of diagnostics and vaccines. The team was unable to visit UVRI. Both the United Kingdom and the CDC operate laboratories on site, primarily related to the human immunodeficiency virus. A BSL-3 laboratory is on site with funding and training provided by CDC. The team was unable to determine unequivocally whether the laboratory had received final certification and was fully functioning. Information was unavailable on UVRI laboratory diagnostic capacity, NIC activities, or triage procedures for suspected human or avian influenza virus specimens and samples. In a later discussion with the Commissioner of Health, human resources were said to be the greatest UVRI need.

Conclusions

The site visit team felt that there were significant and appropriate opportunities in Uganda for the expansion of influenza surveillance activities by USAMRU-K. At the time of the site visit USAMRU-K staff members were working with Makarere University and the Uganda Walter Reed Project to identify and assess laboratory facilities to manage samples from the projects under proposal. It is crucial for in-country relationships that USAMRU-K ensure that Uganda's principal partners (WHO, FAO, CDC) are fully informed of discussions with the MoH.

RECOMMENDATION 6-6. In order to maximize the AI/PI funds in Uganda, USAMRU-K should explore all options, including UVRI, in developing influenza virus diagnostic capacity within Uganda to ensure optimal use of national and external resources, promote collaboration among all sectors, and maximize potential for sustainability.

USAMRU-K Collaborations in Uganda

The National Plan of Action for Preparedness and Response to Avian Influenza in Uganda was released in April 2006. The Plan was developed by the Avian Influenza National Task Force (NTF), which was co-chaired by the commissioners of the MoH and the MAAIF and whose membership included an additional 14 members representing other relevant ministries and development partners. FAO and WHO provided technical support. The plan assesses readiness, assigns responsibilities, guides response preparations, and includes timelines and estimated costs. The major challenges to full implementation of the plan are limited financial and human resources.

Conclusions

The existence of a well-documented national plan, the inclusion of the Ugandan Ministry of Health and Environment, the sharing of personnel between the MoH and Makerere University, and the established programs of both MUWRP and CDC provide a unique opportunity for collaborative influenza surveillance activities in Uganda. Details of such collaborative activities remain to be worked out.

REFERENCES

Bulimo, W. 2007. *The influenza surveillance program at USAMRU-Kenya*. PowerPoint presentation given during site visit on March 13, 2007. Kisumu, Kenya.

DoD-GEIS (Department of Defense Global Emerging Infections System). 2007a. *U.S. Army Medical Research Unit-Kenya.* http://www.geis.fhp.osd.mil/GEIS/Training/USAMRU-K.asp (accessed June 12, 2007).

DoD-GEIS. 2007b. *Department of Defense influenza surveillance sites worldwide, 2007* (unpublished).

IOM (Institute of Medicine). 2001. *Perspectives on the Department of Defense Global Emerging Infections Surveillance and Response System: A program review.* Washington, DC: National Academy Press.

Kenya Red Cross Society. 2006. *Kenya: Avian influenza.* http://www.kenyaredcross.org/UserFiles/File/avian_influenza06.pdf (accessed September 5, 2007).

Limbaso, S. 2007. *Avian influenza: Kenya migratory bird study overview.* PowerPoint presentation given during site visit on March 13, 2007. Kisumu, Kenya.

Schnabel, D. 2007. *The Global Emerging Infectious Disease Surveillance and Response System at USAMRU-Kenya.* PowerPoint presentation given during site visit on March 12, 2007. Kisumu, Kenya.

USAMRU-K. 2007a. *Flu budget* (unpublished).

USAMRU-K. 2007b. *Sample surge capacity plan at USAMRU-K* (unpublished).

USAMRU-K. 2007c. *Lab summary report* (unpublished).

Wabwire-Mangen, F. 2007. *Proposed influenza surveillance project (Uganda).* PowerPoint presentation given during site visit on March 15, 2007. Kampala, Uganda.

WHO (World Health Organization). 2007a. *H5N1 avian influenza: Timeline of major events.* http://www.who.int/csr/disease/avian_influenza/Timeline_2007_03_20.pdf (accessed July 30, 2007).

WHO. 2007b. *Cumulative number of confirmed human cases of avian influenza A/(H5N1) reported to WHO.* http://www.who.int/csr/disease/avian_influenza/country/cases_table_2007_07_25/en/index.html (accessed July 30, 2007).

LIST OF CONTACTS

DoD-GEIS USAMRU-K Assessment: Kenya and Uganda

Kenya

Wallace Bulimo, U.S. Army Medical Research Unit Kenya/National Influenza Center
Margaret Koech, U.S. Army Medical Research Unit Kenya
Dr. Samson Limbaso, U.S. Army Medical Research Unit Kenya
COL Sam Martin, U.S. Army Medical Research Unit Kenya
Bernhards Ogutu, U.S. Army Medical Research Unit Kenya /Kenya Medical Research Institute
Duke Omariba, U.S. Army Medical Research Unit Kenya
Dr. Mark Polhemus, U.S. Army Medical Research Unit Kenya
Fred Sawe, U.S. Army Medical Research Unit Kenya
Capt. David Schnabel, U.S. Army Medical Research Unit Kenya
John Waitumbi, U.S. Army Medical Research Unit Kenya
Dr. Doug Walsh, U.S. Army Medical Research Unit Kenya
Samuel Sinei, Walter Reed Project, Kericho, Kenya
Dr. Phillip Muthoka, Kenyan Ministry of Health

Uganda

Leigh Anne Eller, Makerere University/Walter Reed Project
David Guwatudde, Makerere University/Walter Reed Project
Monica Millard, Makerere University/Walter Reed Project
Arthur Natwijuka, Makerere University/Walter Reed Project
Dr. Denis Byarugaba, Makerere University
Dr. Fred Wabwire-Mangen, Makerere University
Osman Lukwago-Luswa, Makerere University, Institute of Public Health
Lukwago Luswa, Makerere University, Institute of Public Health
Merlin Robb, Henry M. Jackson Foundation
Winyi Kaboyo, Ugandan Ministry of Health
Sam Okware, Ugandan Ministry of Health
Edison Mworozi, Mulago Hospital
Achilles Byaruhanga, Nature Uganda

SCHEDULE OF EVENTS
DoD-GEIS USAMRU-K Assessment

Kisumu, Kenya, and Kampala, Uganda
Participants: Dr. Walter R. Dowdle
Dr. Myron M. Levine
J. Alice Nixon
March 12-16, 2007

Monday, March 12, 2007

0915-0930	**Introduction and Initial Briefing**
0930-1000	**Overview of USAMRU-K** Col. Sam Martin
1045-1045	**Overview of USAMRU-K GEIS program** Capt. David Schnabel
1100-1100	Tea
1130-1130	**Overview of USAMRU-K Kisumu** Col. Doug Walsh
1130-1200	**Acute Febrile Illness protocol** Lt. Col. Mark Polhemus
1200-1300	**Tour Kondele facilities**
1300-1345	Travel to Kombewa
1345-1500	**Overview of Flu program and CDC-International Emerging Infections Program (IEIP)**
1530-1530	**Briefing on Influenza outbreak in Kombewa**
1600-1600	**Tour Kombewa town or district hospital**
1800-1800	Return to hotel

Tuesday, March 13, 2007

0900-1000	**Tour Kericho District Hospital and overview of USAMU-K Kericho program** Dr. Fred Sawe
1200-1200	**Overview of USAMRU-K GEIS flu program** Dr. Wallace Bulimo
1315-1315	**Overview of Migratory Bird Surveillance Project** Dr. Samson Limbaso
1315-1400	**Tour Clinical Trial Center**
1400-1530	**Tour factory**
1730-1730	Return to hotel

Wednesday, March 14, 2007

0900-1600	Travel to Kampala, Uganda

Thursday, March 15, 2007

0900-1030	**Introductions and presentation of Uganda Influenza Work Plan**
1030-1200	**Courtesy visits** Chairman of AI/PI Task Force Makarere University School of Veterinary Medicine Mulago Hospital Outpatient Clinic Makarere University Walter Reed Project (MUWRP)
facilities	
1630-1630	**Field site visit to Kayunga District Hospital**
1700-1700	**Summary of day's events**
1700-	Return to hotel

Friday, March 16, 2007

0930-1130	**Informal discussions and site visit wrap-up**
1130-1230	**Final out-brief**
1230-1700	Lunch and free time
1700-	Departure

7

Naval Medical Research Center Detachment Peru Avian and Pandemic Influenza Activities

The Naval Medical Research Center Detachment Peru (NMRCD), formerly known as the Naval Medical Research Institute Detachment, was established in Lima in 1983 through an agreement between the surgeons general of the Peruvian and U.S. navies, with the concurrence of the U.S. Department of State and the Peruvian Ministry of Foreign Affairs (IOM, 2001). The agreement established a cooperative medical research program to study infectious diseases of interest to both parties. NMRCD is a field detachment of its parent command, the Naval Medical Research Center (NMRC) in Forest Glen, Maryland. Historically, NMRCD has focused on applied research in support of its medical mission. Its past research focus provides a strong framework for the U.S. Department of the Defense Global Emerging Infections Surveillance and Response System (DoD-GEIS) focus on surveillance and response capacity. NMRCD projects receive funding from numerous sources, including the Military Infectious Disease Research Program, the U.S. Department of Defense Southern Command (SOUTHCOM), and DoD-GEIS.

NMRCD is the sole DoD overseas medical research unit in the Western Hemisphere, and it serves a critical role in the DoD-GEIS global network of surveillance and response for emerging infectious diseases. Peru's relative proximity to the continental United States and the frequent commerce and travel between North and South America give this unit an important role in infectious diseases surveillance, particularly as it relates to the biosecurity of the United States (IOM, 2001).

NMRCD now has 230 staff members (15 U.S. military and civilian

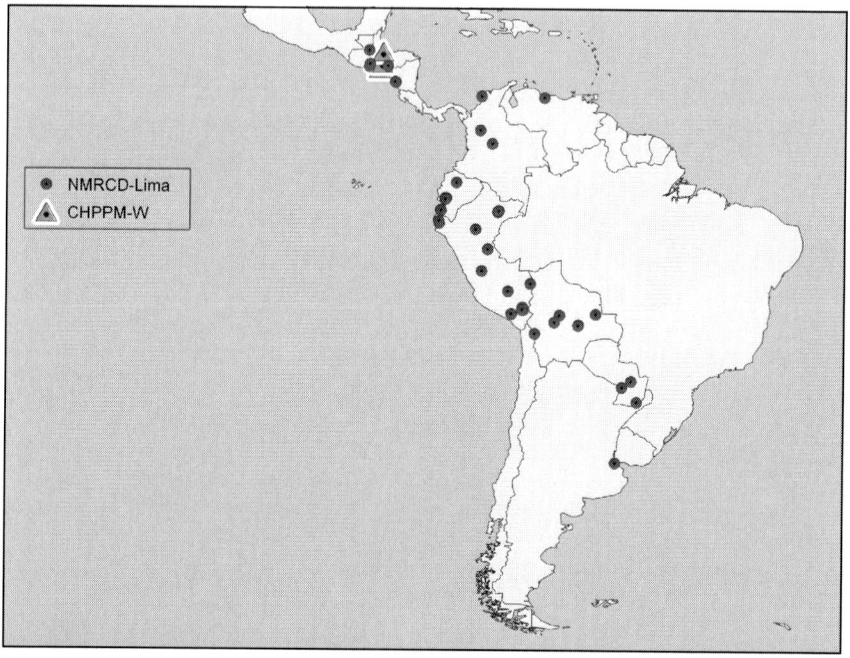

FIGURE 7-1 DoD's regional presence in influenza surveillance (Latin America), 2007.
SOURCE: DoD-GEIS, 2007b.

employees and contractors, 207 Peruvians, and 8 Venezuelans and Bolivians). Most staff are based at a 37,000-square-foot laboratory and animal care facility on the Peruvian naval hospital compound in metropolitan Lima (DoD-GEIS, 2007a). This facility contains three biosafety level 3 (BSL-3) laboratories, including one dedicated to animal investigations. NMRCD also has a new 5,000-square-foot facility on the base of the Peruvian Navy clinic in Iquitos, Peru. The mission of the detachment includes support for vaccine and drug development, evaluation of rapid diagnostics, and surveillance of emerging and re-emerging infectious diseases. The programs and collaborations of NMRCD extend through most of the countries of South and Central America (see Figure 7-1).

The DoD-GEIS program at NMRCD is in alignment with the strategic goals of the overall DoD-GEIS mission as described in the recent five-year plan for the years 2005-2009. DoD-GEIS has identified the following goals as integral to its mission in South America: outbreak response preparation, detection, investigation, microbial agent identification, and communicable disease control and prevention. NMRCD has addressed these goals with its fiscal year 2006 projects, including influenza surveillance and detection, response and readiness, systems research, development and integration, public health capacity building, and training.

A site visit team of the Institute of Medicine (IOM) Committee for the Assessment of DoD-GEIS Influenza Surveillance and Response Programs visited NMRCD from March 4-9, 2007.[1] A list of the people met and interviewed and the itinerary followed can be found at the end of this chapter.

MANAGEMENT AND PLANNING

Staffing

In addition to the administrative sections and the standard research laboratory operating committees, the organization of the laboratory includes seven programmatic science sections: bacteriology, emerging infectious diseases, entomology, parasitology, virology, training, and the Iquitos lab. The leadership is provided by the 13 U.S. scientists, administrators, and technicians, including three Navy physicians, one Army veterinarian, five Navy Ph.D. scientists, one Ph.D. Public Health Service epidemiologist from the Centers for Disease Control and Prevention (CDC), one civilian epidemiologist, and one entomologist. The Peruvian staff includes many highly trained professionals, including physicians, scientists, a veterinarian, and technicians. These Peruvian scientists and administrators provide a large measure of continuity. While the U.S. staff members tend to turn over every several years, many of the civilian staff have been employed at NMRCD for multiple rotations of U.S. staff. This continuity serves a critical role in allowing sustainable programming, especially for ongoing projects which cannot be completed within the tour of a U.S. principal investigator.

A hallmark of NMRCD is that there is extensive cross-disciplinary collaboration between the various science sections. DoD-GEIS appears to be fully integrated across the scientific directorates within the unit. Fieldwork done by the emerging infections section is complemented by the laboratory capabilities of the virology section, and personnel from the training section strengthen the capability for fieldwork. A recent Fogarty International Center training grant benefited not only NMRCD but also many of its external collaborators.

A representative from CDC has brought to NMRCD his extensive experience as a field epidemiologist in outbreak investigation. His tight

---

[1]Prior to the committee's visit to NMRCD, the laboratory staff provided the committee with detailed background information on NMRCD and the pandemic/avian influenza activities they were supporting. These materials are available from the IOM in the Public Access File.

links with CDC experts also facilitate strong interagency communications. Although this CDC representative leads the outbreak investigation section, he also plays a central role in influenza surveillance and associated forms of outreach to Peruvian collaborators. The influenza surveillance program also makes good use of the technical field expertise of a staff veterinarian.

Technology and Information Management

NMRCD employs state-of-the-art tools for communications and information management. In addition to a well-organized in-house data processing center, NMRCD has pioneered in Latin America several innovative information technology systems; one example is ALERTA, which is used for reportable disease surveillance of Peruvian military populations, including virtually all elements of the Peruvian Navy. Employing an effective mix of appropriate technologies including cell phones, radios, and the Internet, this system allows rapid surveillance from remote jungle areas and Pacific-based ships. The system's suitability has been well evaluated according to CDC-recommended criteria. NMRCD has also adapted the NAMRU-2 Early Warning Outbreak Response System (EWORS) for syndromic surveillance in Peru. The detachment has also been able to make use of current U.S. military remote-sensing mapping photos in the course of outbreak investigations.

NMRCD is also efficiently connected to collaborators through excellent Internet connectivity, cell phones, and personal digital assistants. As one might imagine, connectivity is less robust for some partner organizations in Peru. In particular, the Ministry of Health Directorate of General Epidemiology (DGE) noted a serious need for an integrated real-time national public health information-management system to foster hierarchical communications between the local, regional, and national epidemiology and public health laboratory authorities. The DGE has a slower hierarchical system of reportable disease reporting called NOTI. NMRCD may be able to make a valuable contribution in helping to transfer insights from U.S. public health information-management systems. In addition, through its extensive regional collaborations, NMRCD may also be able to identify the best approaches to information management and foster exchange of relevant information-management system tools from other countries in the region. Perhaps through partnerships with the U.S. Agency for International Development (USAID), Pan American Health Organization (PAHO), and other technical and donor organizations, NMRCD and DoD-GEIS can play a useful role in fostering the development of the type of an effective real-time information system that will save critical time in an outbreak. It would seem that individual "home grown" information-management systems would not be the most effective or cost-effective way of implementing the type of communication tools central to multi-agency outbreak detection and response. In addition, NMRCD is developing a Web-based software program to provide real-time surveillance data to the DoD, the wider U.S. government, and the global public health community.

Conclusions

Communication with the DoD-GEIS Headquarters in Silver Spring has been effective, and at the time of the IOM team visit it had recently increased. The addition of strong, experienced staff at DoD-GEIS in Silver Spring has been clearly of benefit. Regularly scheduled telephone or video conferences with these DoD-GEIS partners would help to exchange information and experiences with respect to pandemic influenza preparedness.

RECOMMENDATION 7-1. NMRCD should continue to work to increase information sharing with both the DoD-GEIS headquarters staff and staff at other overseas laboratories.

While the site visit team found the avian influenza/pandemic influenza (AI/PI) activities being conducted at NMRCD to be well planned and executed, NMRCD could contribute more significantly to the evaluation of national influenza preparedness. For example, tabletop simulations may help NMRCD, the U.S. Department of Health and Human Services (HHS), and the U.S. Department of Agriculture (USDA) direct future investments of pandemic preparedness funding for Peru.

RECOMMENDATION 7-2. NMRCD should support additional tabletop simulation exercises in which NMRCD has the potential to identify areas of the Peruvian plan that need strengthening.

SURVEILLANCE

Human Surveillance

The DoD-GEIS-sponsored ALERTA surveillance system for monitoring reportable diseases in the Peruvian Navy has been extended to the Peruvian Army. The Navy now has 50 reporting units covering 97.5 percent of the Navy. An ALERTA training program has conducted 47 courses and has trained a total of 877 persons, and ALERTA reports increased from 3,700 in 2003 to approximately 25,000 in 2005 (NMRCD, 2006). There are plans to use SOUTHCOM funding to extend this surveillance system to the Colombian military. It would be desirable to establish a link between ALERTA clinical reports and laboratory-based surveillance reports.

The NAMRU-2 EWORS syndromic surveillance system has been successfully implemented in Lima and Tumbes. These electronic surveillance systems have identified two recent influenza B outbreaks involving approximately 80 people (NMRCD, 2006). The head of the surveillance unit presented an excellent systematic evaluation of these systems using the CDC-recommended schema for the evaluation of surveillance systems.

NMRCD has a long-standing febrile syndrome surveillance protocol under DoD-GEIS. NMRCD's surveillance study, performed primarily with the General Office of Epidemiology in Lima and the National Institute of Health in Lima, is supported by approximately 10 additional collaborating institutions in Peru and the U.S. This prospective observational study of febrile disease syndromes in Peru began in May 2000 and will end in 2008. Involved in this study are approximately 20,400 subjects, including the 10,000 individuals who were enrolled in the study's first five years, an additional 2,000 individuals being recruited through active surveillance and 7,200 by passive surveillance, as well as 1,200 Peruvian military personnel. As described in their May 2006 protocol, the sample size was calculated to study about 400 patients per study site per year, for a total of about 30 patients per month at each of the sites. Currently about 64 clinics and hospitals (military and civilian) participate in febrile syndrome surveillance, and all can provide rapid diagnosis for influenza.

The protocol focuses on patients presenting to selected health services or detected during the active surveillance with fever (oral) greater or equal to 38°C, 7 days or less in duration, accompanied by one or more of the following: headache, muscle, ocular and/or joint pain, generalized fatigue, cough, nausea/vomiting, sore throat, rhinnorhea, difficulty breathing, diarrhea, bloody stools, jaundiced, dizziness, disoriented, stiff neck, petechiae, ecchymoses, bleeding gum and/or nose. Only individuals five years of age or older are included, unless hemorrhagic manifestations are present. Acute and convalescent blood specimens are drawn, and a throat swab is obtained from individuals presenting with an influenza-like illness characterized primarily by a fever, generalized fatigue, sore throat and rhinorrhea.

With the help of AI/PI funds this long-standing surveillance protocol has been successfully adapted to incorporate influenza surveillance. This surveillance approach is now being extended to the Colombian Army, National Police, and Navy as well as to two Army sites in Ecuador. NMRCD provides salaries for approximately ten physicians to operate this network (NMRCD, 2006). The influenza surveillance capabilities include isolation from nasopharyngeal swabs, polymerase chain reaction (PCR), and sequencing at NMRCD. Good primers are in hand for human influenza, but more effective primers for avian influenza need to be identified. With the AI/PI funding, diagnostic capacity has been extended to include a wider range of respiratory agents. Some sites send weekly shipments to Lima, and other locations forward samples on a monthly basis. Reporting to the ministries of health, participating physicians, and the Air Force Institute for Operational Health (AFIOH) in San Antonio, Texas, takes place on a monthly basis (AFIOH, 2004). Critical results are reported directly after sequence confirmation. Continued expansion of diagnostic capabilities is planned and will include coronaviruses. Avian virus surveillance will also be expanded. Consideration is being given to expanding efforts to other countries such as Suriname. Screening for antiviral resistance is not a current capability. The fiscal year 2006 AI/PI funding allowed the addition of about 40 new surveillance sites.

The NMRCD scope of activities covers a wide range, including molecular biology, descriptive epidemiology, and social science efforts. The social science-oriented surveillance has tracked knowledge, attitude, and behavior concerning influenza among occupationally at-risk workers. A Peruvian social scientist will be involved in addressing risk communication issues. NMRCD collaborates with many partners, including the CDC, MoH, USAID, PAHO, DGE, and the Instituto Nacional de Salud. Capacity building is central to the program.

Animal Surveillance

In addition to human surveillance, the NMRCD program extends to avian influenza. It is a participant in the Global Avian Influenza Network Surveillance, managed by the World Wildlife Conservation Society at the Bronx Zoo (NMRCD, 2006). This network focuses on surveillance of dead and dying birds in coastal areas as well as on droppings from closely observed migratory birds along coastal lagoons.

The self-assessment of NMRCD is that their efforts are weakest in the area of animal surveillance. One of the surveillance initiatives planned to address this deficit is active surveillance of influenza-like illness in chicken farm workers using an electronic surveillance approach. Surveillance of workers in the large mixed live bird markets of Lima is also under consideration. Both of these activities were deemed to be of value to establishing current influenza patterns. Another plan is to study different strategies to optimize reporting within electronic surveillance systems.

Conclusions

The site visit team found that NMRCD has a suite of innovative surveillance systems that benefit from not only DoD-GEIS AI/PI funds but also DoD-GEIS core funding as well as leveraging from associations with CDC, the Fogarty International Center, USAID, and SOUTHCOM.

RECOMMENDATION 7-3. NMRCD should consider expanding its surveillance activities to include populations at high risk of contracting avian influenza, including poultry farm workers, live bird market workers, and recruits in military training camps.

LABORATORY

NMRCD possesses three BSL-3 containment laboratories. Two are located in the main laboratory complex, and a third is located in the animal care facility laboratory. If required, this latter unit could be modified into two separate BSL-3 laboratories rather easily. For influenza testing the laboratory has both conventional and real-time PCR capability as well as the ability to do immunofluroescence testing. Conventional virus culture is done using various cell lines that are maintained in the laboratory. All laboratories are inspected twice annually and a Peruvian technologist trained in the United States certifies safety hoods annually. Renovations and upgrades to the laboratory are being made on a continuing basis to enhance its capability and efficiency. The ability to operate at the BSL-3 enhanced level could be achieved by adding shower-out facilities.

The NMRCD virology program has the necessary human influenza A primers to identify any isolated virus, including the full complement of hemagglutinins, key neuraminidases, and matrix protein. The laboratory is collaborating with the CDC to increase its complement of primers for avian influenza. This should hopefully reduce some of the delays that have been experienced in the characterizing of avian influenza types.

The laboratory currently has two sequencers, a 16-column and a 4-column unit. Consideration is currently being given to trading the 4-column unit up to another 16-column unit to increase sequencing capacity. While the current sequencing capacity is generally adequate for the present workload, two 16-column units would provide a significant enhancement in surge capacity.

The laboratory role of NMRCD in AI/PI surveillance in Peru and the Andean Region is of crucial importance. From 1999-2004 AFIOH performed all influenza virus identifications. While the technical and scientific support provided by AFIOH was excellent, the current ability of NMRCD to perform in-house testing has greatly decreased the turnaround time required to report test results to submitters. This in turn has encouraged clinical sites to place much greater value on participation in surveillance activities.

At the present time NMRCD does not have separate laboratory suites for the testing and identification of avian and human influenza isolates. The current laboratory layout will allow for necropsy of dead birds and specimen collection in the BSL-3 unit in the animal care facility laboratory.

Specimens then are tested by immunofluorescence (IF) and PCR in the same area used for the testing of human isolates located in the main laboratory complex. As the World Health Organization (WHO) recommends that clinical specimens from humans and from swine or birds should never be processed in the same laboratory, consideration should be given to how this might be best accomplished (WHO, 2007). At a minimum, any option chosen to separate human and animal isolations would require the development of additional IF/PCR capability in which only AI specimens would be tested, either at NMRCD or possibly at another collaborating Peruvian sites, such as the Servicio Nacional de Sanidad Agraria (SENASA). It is recommended that NMRCD propose this additional capability in future funding requests.

Conclusions

The site visit team found NMRCD's plans to improve the laboratory worthwhile. These plans included the extension of diagnostic capabilities and avian influenza surveillance, the addition of capability for coronaviruses and non-H5N1 avian viruses, and the expansion of surveillance efforts to additional countries.

RECOMMENDATION 7-4. In conjunction with improved sharing of facilities for testing avian viruses at SENASA, NMRCD should develop mechanisms to enable testing of avian and human influenza isolates in separate laboratory facilities and plan to obtain resources to expand its BSL-3 laboratory, including showering-out facilities.

RESPONSE CAPACITY

Outbreak Investigation

Outbreak response has been central to NMRCD. NMRCD is well positioned to respond to influenza outbreaks, as evidenced from its experiences in 2006-2007 when it responded to outbreaks of plague, yellow fever, diarrhea, cyclospora, undifferentiated febrile syndrome, Venezuelan equine encephalitis, mumps, dengue, rabies, and influenza. The recent posting of a representative from CDC extends this capacity considerably. NMRCD is building a considerable network and capacity for both surveillance of and response to outbreaks.

The training unit has sponsored 33 iterations of the NMRCD outbreak-investigation course. Since 2002 an avian influenza case study has been included in the course. Over 1,300 trainees from 14 countries have been trained over the past five years. Other institutions in Latin American have been adapting the course to local needs. These courses have been conducted in collaboration with PAHO, CDC, and USAID. Reports have been received on 248 outbreaks.

Surge Capacity

As part of the committee's data gathering, NMRCD was asked to estimate the number of samples it would be able to process in the following four scenarios: routine operation (baseline); an altered algorithm, testing only for influenza A and H5; PCR testing to amplify only one specific gene from H5; and, finally, not only making these other modifications but also arranging to perform tests 24 hours per day, seven days a week.

According to information provided to the committee, NMRCD routinely does cell culture isolation on all respiratory specimens. The influenza isolates are typed as A or B by this process and are then genotyped by reverse transcription polymerase chain reaction (RT-PCR) and sequencing. Under normal conditions approximately 100 specimens per week are processed by cell culture isolation. Specimens in transport media are not usually screened by RT-PCR because the sensitivity of RT-PCR is slightly less than that of cell culture isolation. Under normal conditions, 200 specimens per week can be processed by RT-PCR (NMRCD, 2007).

Under 24-hours–a-day, seven-days-a-week conditions at NMRCD, 300 specimens per week can be processed by cell culture isolation and 1,000 specimens per week can be processed by RT-PCR (NMRCD, 2007).

Conclusions

Although there have not been any reported cases of H5 highly pathogenic avian influenza in Peru or South America in general, NMRCD does have experience in infectious disease outbreak investigations as well as a surge capacity plan in the event that an avian outbreak does occur.

CAPACITY BUILDING

NMRCD Laboratory Capacity

NMRCD has been doing respiratory disease surveillance since 1996, but AI supplemental funds have allowed for the expansion and improvement of these programs. In the past, NMRCD relied on AFIOH to conduct the viral isolation and identification of samples collected in Peru, which led to delays of several months in receiving the results. Using supplemental funds NMRCD has increased its capacity to detect influenza with cell culture, real-time PCR, and gene-sequencing capabilities. This capacity allows NMRCD to return results to providers quickly, keeping collaborators engaged and patients satisfied with the results.

In addition to the NMRCD laboratory capability having been increased, the number of sites from which NMRCD actively collects respiratory specimens has increased as well. Samples are collected from sites in 10 countries throughout South and Central America. Peru has the most active sites with 25; other sites are located in Argentina, Bolivia, Colombia, Ecuador, El Salvador, Honduras, Nicaragua, Paraguay, and Venezuela.

NMRCD Training Activities

NMRCD puts a strong emphasis on training. The training unit has sponsored 33 iterations of the NMRCD outbreak investigation course. Since 2002 an avian influenza case study has been included in the course. Over 1,300 trainees from 14 countries have been trained over the past five years. Other institutions in Latin America have been adapting the course to local needs. These courses have been conducted in collaboration with PAHO, CDC, and USAID. NMRCD also has a Fogarty Center Training grant that funds Peruvians from NMRCD and other organizations to attend the Johns Hopkins Bloomberg School of Public Health summer session (two per year), to attend the one-year MPH program at the Uniformed Services University of the Health Sciences (USUHS), and to obtain doctoral training in the United States. The grant will also be used to help initiate a master's level program at Cayetano-Heredia University. NMRCD has also made a commitment to offering training seminars through the download of webcasts from the United States and has sponsored a number of very well attended sessions on various laboratory practices.

In addition to outbreak training, NMRCD has provided a number of courses in the conduct of research, bioethics, data analysis, and epidemiology. Students from many institutions based in the United States have been rotating regularly through NMRCD. These include USUHS, the University of Washington, the University of Iowa, Johns Hopkins University, Emory University, Tulane University, Kansas State University, and the State University of New York at Stony Brook. Considering the demand for training at NMRCD, the successes to date, and the need for wider and deeper human networks to address emerging infections including AI/PI, further investment in physical classroom and teaching laboratory facilities as well as human infrastructure to support training is encouraged. NMRCD is clearly a suitable focal point for U.S. investments in epidemiological and laboratory capacity building in Latin America.

Conclusions

NMRCD's track record for pre-service and in-service training to U.S. and Peruvian students and practitioners is impressive. It has developed a well-received outbreak investigation course that has built a wide network of contacts across Peru and Latin America.

RECOMMENDATION 7-5. NMRCD should continue to support in-house and webcast training in epidemiological surveillance and laboratory methods. Outbreak response should receive additional emphasis, including Peru's Field Epidemiology Training Program.

COLLABORATION AND COORDINATION

Host Country Government

NMRCD is clearly engaged with a wide range of national and regional influenza-related committees and organizations involved with avian and human influenza surveillance and response. NMRCD's network is active and wide, encompassing not only the ministries of health and agriculture but also Peruvian Army and Navy medical surveillance channels.

The NMRCD influenza program has established substantial networks with relevant entities in the Peruvian government, including the Instituto Nacional de Salud (INS), the Directorate de Epidemiologia General, and SENASA. Peru manages its national influenza-preparedness program through three committees: an executive committee chaired by the Vice Minister of Health, a committee of technical support, and a national multisectoral committee. NMRCD is a recognized advisor to these entities. Ironically, the detachment may also help serve as a bridge between human and animal health-oriented elements of the Peruvian government, which don't seem to have yet established close communications on influenza issues. Peru has a detailed and thoughtful pandemic influenza-preparedness plan on paper based on 1999 and 2005 WHO guidance. It would appear, however, that the plan is not well-resourced. Issues such as the ability to diagnose cases and institute effective infection control in the face of a pandemic are of concern. The Ministry of Agriculture's laboratory, SENASA, has a mandate from the Food and Agricultural Organization and the World Organization for Animal Health to do animal surveillance for influenza, but resources to conduct this surveillance are quite limited. Resources are also limited for the INS influenza laboratory, staffed by only three persons, to process more than a handful of the specimens that NMRCD shares with it. Independent collection of specimens by the INS influenza laboratory is compromised in a number of locations around Peru by issues surrounding the cold chain, the series of low-temperature facilities used for storing samples. These limitations have prompted the INS to focus on surveillance in intensive care units, whereas the NMRCD collects specimens primarily from primary care settings. A unified national influenza-surveillance database combining data from the NMRCD and Peruvian government laboratories would seem desirable.

As noted above, NMRCD collaborates with a number of Peruvian government agencies on influenza surveillance. These agencies lack resources in many cases. Though they have willing professionals, obstacles such as unreliable cold chains hinder the amount of work that can be done. NMRCD laboratory space and other resources are available to the INS to support influenza virus isolation. The laboratory leadership appeared to understand and be sensitive to the potential challenges associated with the large resource gap for influenza between NMRCD and the INS. In order to strengthen collective Peruvian diagnostic capacity to characterize influenza viruses, NMRCD should continue to work collaboratively with other laboratory resources in country, including offers of assistance, resource sharing, and a common database.

Multilateral Agencies

Though NMRCD has strong relationships with Peruvian government entities involved in influenza surveillance and response, it is clearly in the position to be a leading source of U.S. government assistance if AI/PI emerges as a problem in the region. NMRCD has applied in the past for designation as a WHO Collaborating Center for Emerging Infections. It is reported that despite the passage of more than a year, the application has not been forwarded from PAHO in Washington, D.C., to the WHO in Geneva. To better position NMRCD to provide expert reference-level surveillance and response assistance to other countries of South and Central America, WHO Collaborating Center status should be aggressively pursued, perhaps with the support of leadership from other U.S. government departments such as the State Department and HHS. The head of the PAHO country office in Peru suggested that NMRCD solicit the active support of ministers of health in other Andean countries to request that status for NMRCD.

U.S. Government Agencies

The officer-in-charge of the NMRCD is a participating member of the U.S. embassy country team under the leadership of the U.S. ambassador to Peru. It was clear that NMRCD has the strong support of the U.S. ambassador and that the U.S. ambassador specifically appreciates and values the role of the NMRDC in strengthening avian and pandemic influenza surveillance in Peru and the region. He has supported relevant increases in staffing levels and has, from his position, successfully encouraged Peruvian officials to address the global threat of avian and pandemic influenza. Within the embassy, NMRCD is seen as a valuable source of consultation with respect to USDA investments in controlling avian influenza in the region. NMRCD is also well connected to the USAID section at the embassy. The overall fiscal year 2006 operating budget of the detachment was $10,025,169.28. The DoD-GEIS core budget was $1.34 million. The fiscal year 2006 AI/PI supplement brought $1.74 million to the laboratory. For fiscal year 2007, the desired AI/PI budget is $2.20 million, of which $750,000 has been received to date.

HHS has provided $825,000 in funding to Peru for pandemic influenza preparedness, of which 80 percent was earmarked for epidemiologic and laboratory strengthening. NMRCD has offered to help the Peruvian government with various aspects, such as provision of a database to help with monitoring national influenza trends and improving diagnostic capacities at the INS. One of the main challenges for the Peruvian government influenza surveillance network is the cold chain needed to preserve specimens collected around the country. NMRCD has offered use of its ultra-low-temperature freezers around the country as well as assistance with biosafety issues. The detachment has also offered other electronic surveillance technologies to supplement those of the government.

NMRCD has an open relationship with the USAID program in Peru, though the USAID commitment to influenza in Peru is not major. Based on the observations of the site visit team, NMRCD is respected by USAID as an important builder of regional capacity. Perhaps surprisingly, a senior Peruvian USAID staffer said that NMRCD has brought consistency to some programs in the face of turnover in the Peruvian government. As the Peruvian governmental health care system becomes more decentralized, USAID sees capacity building as much needed.

The assignment of a representative from CDC to NMRCD illustrates that there is a serious commitment, backed by human resources, to maintain collaboration between the DoD and CDC. The representative's tight links with CDC experts also facilitate strong interagency communications.

In addition to partnering effectively with the HHS, NMRCD has leveraged DoD humanitarian assistance funds to improve regional surveillance. A very strong working relationship was evident between NMRCD and the office of the military assistance group at the U.S. embassy.

Conclusions

NMRCD is a critical national and regional resource for avian influenza/pandemic influenza surveillance and response as well as for addressing other emerging infectious diseases. It has established a strong reputation in the region and is well positioned to support emerging infections surveillance, response, and capacity building. It is well integrated into several governmental and multisectoral committees formed to prepare for the Peruvian national response. Though perhaps less practical, it could also play a valuable role for other Andean countries. Host countries appreciate its role and for the most part trust its leaders in sensitive matters. Without a doubt many Latin American countries will turn to NMRCD for its expertise and capabilities in the face of a national emerging infections crisis, such as an outbreak of avian or epidemic influenza. A renewed drive for WHO Collaborating Center status should be undertaken with the support of other ministers of health in the Andean Region.

NMRCD has much deeper resources for influenza work than are available to Peruvian government counterparts. It needs to continue to be sensitive to the potential unintended consequences of this resource imbalance so as to not allow the collateral weakening of Peruvian government capacities if providers preferentially turn to NMRCD for diagnostic support.

RECOMMENDATION 7-6. A close working relationship, the sharing of facilities, the training of technicians, the sharing of specimens, support for maintenance, support to meet cold-chain needs, and other forms of integration with the INS and SENASA laboratories should continue to be cultivated by NMRCD. A common surveillance database with both NMRCD and INS results would be desirable.

REFERENCES

Air Force Institute for Operational Health (AFIOH). 2004. *DoD global influenza and other respiratory viral pathogens surveillance weekly update week 14 (4 Apr–10 Apr)*. http://www.geis.fhp.osd.mil/GEIS/SurveillanceActivities/Influenza/Reports/influenza_2004-04-04.pdf (accessed September 5, 2007).

DoD-GEIS (Department of Defense Global Emerging Infections System). 2007a. *U.S. Naval Medical Research Center Detachment*. http://www.geis.fhp.osd.mil/GEIS/Training/nmrcd.asp (accessed July 30, 2007).

DoD-GEIS. 2007b. *Department of Defense influenza surveillance sites worldwide, 2007* (unpublished).

IOM (Institute of Medicine). 2001. Perspectives on the Department of Defense Global Emerging Infections Surveillance and Response System: A program review. Washington, DC: The National Academies Press.

NMRCD (U.S. Naval Medical Research Center Detachment). 2006. *Influenza and disease surveillance summary* (unpublished).

NMRCD. 2007. *Surge capacity plan* (unpublished).

WHO (World Health Organization). 2007. *Recommended laboratory tests to identify avian influenza A virus in specimens from humans March 2007*. http://www.who.int/csr/disease/avian_influenza/guidelines/labtestsMarch07web.pdf (accessed August 15, 2007).

LIST OF CONTACTS

DoD-GEIS NMRCD Assessment: Peru

Cmdr. David Blazes, Naval Medical Research Center Detachment, Lima, Peru
Lt. Cmdr. Tadeusz Kochel, Naval Medical Research Center Detachment, Lima, Peru
Andres Lescano, Naval Medical Research Center Detachment, Lima, Peru
Lt. Cmdr. Joel Montgomery, Naval Medical Research Center Detachment, Lima, Peru
Cecilia Mundaca, Naval Medical Research Center Detachment, Lima, Peru
Milagros Salazar Gross, Naval Medical Research Center Detachment, Lima, Peru
Ambassador J. Curtis Struble, U.S. Embassy, Lima Peru
Col. Jeffrey H. Fargo, United States Military Advisory and Assistance Group, Department of Defense, Washington, D.C.
Eugene Philhower, United States Department of Agriculture, Lima, Peru
Michele Russell, United States Agency for International Development, Lima, Peru
Luis Seminario, United States Agency for International Development, Lima, Peru
Twani Ortiz Almeida, Dirección General de Epidemiología, Lima, Peru
Jorge Goméz Benavides, Dirección General de Epidemiología, Lima, Peru
Paúl Pachas Chavez, Dirección General de Epidemiología, Lima, Peru
José Bolarte Espinoza, Dirección General de Epidemiología, Lima, Peru
Gladys Ramírez Prada, Dirección General de Epidemiología, Lima, Peru
Aguiles Vilchez, Dirección General de Epidemiología, Lima, Peru
Roberto Acosta, Servicio Nacional de Sanidad Agraria, Lima, Peru
Roberto Antonio Acosta Galvez, Servicio Nacional de Sanidad Agraria, Lima, Peru
Ysabel Montoya, Servicio Nacional de Sanidad Agraria, Lima, Peru
C. Juan Raul Zegarra Valencia, Servicio Nacional de Sanidad Agraria, Lima, Peru
Carolina Alvarado Dueñas, Dirección General de Salud a las Personas, Lima, Peru
Maria Luz Sotomayor, Dirección General de Salud a las Personas, Lima, Peru
Victor Fiestas Solorzano, Instituto Nacional de Salud, Lima, Peru
Yvonne Torres, Insituto Nacional de Salud, Lima, Peru
José F. Picón Gonzales, Instituto Nacional de Defensa Civil, Lima, Peru

Armando E. Gonzalez, University San Marcos/Johns Hopkins School of Public Health
Manuel Peña, Pan American Health Organization/World Health Organization, Lima, Peru

SCHEDULE OF EVENTS
DoD-GEIS NMRCD Assessment

Lima, Peru
Participants: Dr. James M. Hughes
Dr. K. Mills McNeill
Dr. Patrick Kelley
March 4-10, 2007

Sunday, March 4, 2007

1000-1600	Tour of the city
1900-2000	Dinner

Monday, March 5, 2007

0730-0800	Drive to NMRCD
0815-0915	**Review of Peruvian National Preparedness Plan** Lt. Cmdr. Joel Montgomery, USPHS, Director, Outbreak Investigation and Response Team, Emerging Diseases Program
0915-1000	**Presentation on status of Emerging Infections Program** Cmdr. David Blazes, Director of EDP
1000-1015	Break
1015-1100	**Presentation on electronic surveillance of Influenza** Dr. Cecilia Mundaca, Electronic Surveillance Unit, Emerging Infections Program
1100-1145	**Presentation on training** Andres Lescano
1200-1300	Lunch
1300-1500	**Presentation on virology laboratory** Lt. Cmdr. Tadeusz Kochel, MSC, USN, Director of Virology Program
1500-1630	**Tour of facilities**
1630-1845	Return to hotel
1845-2000	Dinner Virology Department GEIS Team
2000-2030	Return to hotel

Tuesday, March 6, 2007

0800-0810	**Courtesy visit** Eugene Philhower, Foreign Agriculture Service
0815-0845	**Courtesy visit** Col. Jeffrey Fargo, Chief Military Assistance and Advisory Group
0900-0920	**Courtesy visit** Ambassador J. Curtis Struble
0930-1000	**Courtesy visit at health office of USAID** Michele Russell Luis Seminario
1000-1015	**Commissary at American Embassy**
1015-1200	Travel to NMRCD
1200-1330	Lunch
1330-1400	Travel to PAHO
1400-1600	**Meeting** Dr. Manuel Peña, PAHO/WHO Representative
1600-1630	*Return to hotel*

Wednesday, March 7, 2007

1000-1100	**Tour of SENASA**
1200-1300	Lunch
1300-1315	Walk to Dirección General de Epidemiología
1330-1630	**Meeting with Ministry of Health Avian Influenza Working Group** Representatives of MoH, INS, DGE, SENASA
1630-1700	Return to hotel

Thursday, March 8, 2007

0900-1030	**Visit bird site (Pantanos de Villa, Chorrillos)** Cmdr. David Blazes Lt. Cmdr. Joel Montgomery Dr. Milagros Salazar Dr. Armando Gonzales
1030-1200	**Tour San Marcos Veterinary School Laboratory**
1200-1600	Lunch/free time
1600-1630	Return to hotel

Friday, March 9, 2007

0830-2130	Closeout day at NMRCD (?)
2130-2200	Drive to airport

Saturday, March 10, 2007

0035-	Departure

8

Naval Health Research Center San Diego Avian and Pandemic Influenza Activities

The Naval Respiratory Disease Laboratory (NRDL), established in 1996 to perform epidemiological studies and surveillance of respiratory diseases affecting U.S. military personnel, is one of six departments of the Naval Health Research Center (NHRC) in San Diego, California (NHRC, 2006b). NHRC was instrumental in demonstrating increased adenoviral morbidity among basic trainees after loss of vaccine in the late 1990s, and it remains involved in the restoration of the adenovirus vaccine program by supporting current clinical trials at basic training centers (NHRC, 2006b). NHRC has continually expanded its scope of studies and diagnostics during the past decade, with an increased emphasis on influenza surveillance and diagnostics; molecular capabilities in particular have been greatly enhanced. NHRC has become a leading reference laboratory for respiratory disease within the Department of Defense (DoD) (NHRC, 2006b). During fiscal year 2006, NHRC doubled laboratory testing capacity for influenza, began construction of a biosafety level 3 enhanced (BSL-3E) laboratory, and conducted a variety of projects sponsored by the Department of Defense Global Emerging Infections Surveillance and Response System (DoD-GEIS) that contributed to force health protection.

DoD-GEIS AI supplemental funding increased surge capacity in 2006-2007. Five new staff members were added, sample target numbers for each surveillance site were doubled, the frequency of shipments to the NRDL at NHRC was increased, and laboratory equipment was updated or added. The result was more robust surveillance and faster turnaround. More than

2,000 samples were collected and tested during the influenza season of October 2006 through February 2007.

A site visit team of the Institute of Medicine (IOM) Committee for the Assessment of DoD-GEIS Influenza Surveillance and Response Programs visited NHRC on March 26-27, 2007.[1] A list of the people met and interviewed and the itinerary followed can be found at the end of this chapter.

MANAGEMENT AND PLANNING

Administrative support for NRDL is provided by the DoD Center for Deployment Health Research at the time of the IOM review. However, in August of 2007, the Respiratory Disease Laboratory became an independent department at HHRC, Department of Respiratory Diseases Research. DoD-GEIS funding makes up more than 90 percent of the NRDL budget and is used for special projects and capital improvements.

Staffing

NRDL staff is composed of both Navy personnel and civilians. The GEIS-related projects at NRDL are managed by the laboratory director, co-director, and several study coordinators, who receive input from the project staff, including two Ph.D. consultants, a consulting pathologist, epidemiologists, a statistician, 16 full-time technicians, 7 off-site study coordinators, and 5 staff members dedicated to quality assurance and control.

The IOM committee commends the NRDL leadership for devoting both time and personnel to important aspects of diagnostic testing, that is, exploring new and advanced diagnostic platforms and incoming technologies, maintaining a high level of quality control, and being open to new and improved methodologies that promote faster and more accurate test results.

Technology and Information Management

The laboratory information-management system used by the NHRC is an Access-based program designed specifically for the laboratory. The system operates well for the laboratory. Efforts are underway to find a bar-coding system that is compatible with and can be incorporated into the existing systems.

[1]Prior to the committee's visit to NHRC, the laboratory staff provided the committee with detailed background information on NHRC and the pandemic/avian influenza activities it was supporting. These materials were used in the writing of this chapter and are available from the IOM in the Public Access File.

The sequence analysis conducted in this laboratory is of the highest quality. The team at NHRC seems able to utilize the data generated for evaluations of vaccine efficacy, recognizing emerging novel viruses, and evaluations in different areas.

Conclusions

The committee found the NHRC staff proficient at the generation and analysis of high-quality virus and sequence data. They are timely in producing their findings as well as in reporting them back to their clients and collaborating laboratories. The NHRC data would be a tremendous asset to modeling efforts.

SURVEILLANCE

The missions of the NHRC are to conduct epidemiological studies to investigate the health experience of military personnel and their families and to develop and evaluate appropriate health strategies. The stated objectives of NRDL are to help enhance febrile respiratory and influenza surveillance, advance influenza diagnostics, and improve influenza field diagnostics as well as to assist with the coordination of overseas response capabilities, with the early detection of and response to respiratory disease, with enhanced communication within DoD, and with maintaining the health of U.S. military forces worldwide (NHRC, 2006a).

The NRDL initiated febrile respiratory illness (FRI) surveillance for adenovirus in five basic-training sites in 1996 and was accredited by the College of American Pathologists (CAP) in 1997. In 1998 FRI surveillance increased to the present eight sites and expanded to include other viral pathogens: influenza A and B, respiratory syncytial virus, and parainfluenza types 1, 2, and 3 (Faix, 2006). Additional ongoing FRI surveillance includes personnel on board 16 Navy ships deployed worldwide and also civilian populations near the border between the United States and Mexico (Faix, 2006). Each of the three populations presents distinct FRI risks (see Figure 8-1 for a map of NRDL FRI surveillance sites).

Other projects among military trainees include the etiology and epidemiology of pneumonia, characterization of clinical *Streptococcus pyogenes*, and surveillance for *Bordetella pertussis*. Surveillance for antibiotic resistance in invasive *Streptococcus pneumonia* is conducted among DoD beneficiaries. NRDL is currently involved in a collaborative phase 3 study to evaluate the safety, efficacy, and immunogenicity of the vaccines for adenovirus 4 and adenovirus 7. NRDL should consider expanding the current FRI case definition in certain situations to capture influenza illness that

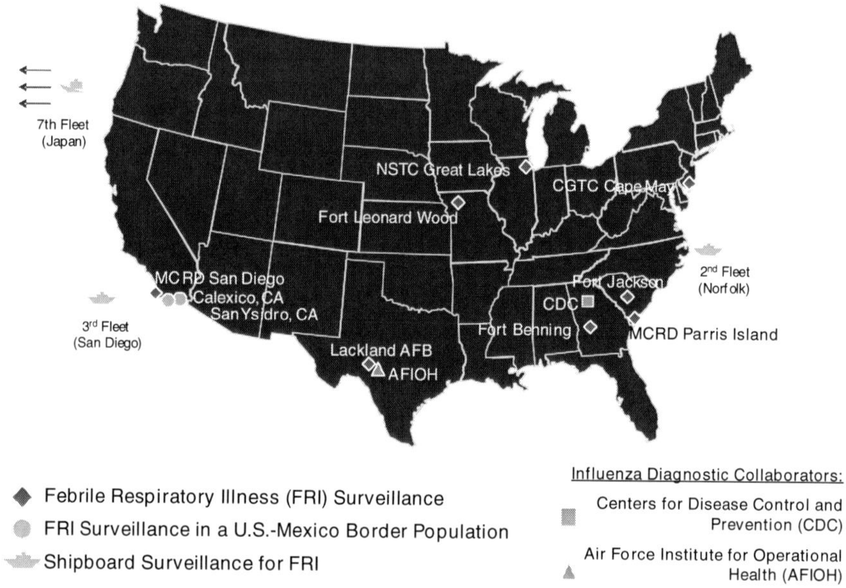

FIGURE 8-1 NHRC influenza surveillance sites and activities, 2006-2007.
SOURCE: Faix, 2006.

could present with different or unusual symptoms, such as conjunctivitis or diarrhea.

FRI Surveillance Among Military Trainees

Surveillance is conducted at eight of the ten DoD U.S. training sites, representing all service branches: the Army (Ft. Jackson, Ft. Leonard Wood, and Ft. Benning), the Navy (Naval Training Center Great Lakes), the Marines (Marine Corps Recruit Depot San Diego and Marine Corps Recruit Depot Parris Island), the Air Force (Lackland Air Force Base), and the Coast Guard (Training Center Cape May). The two training sites not included are Ft. Knox and Ft. Sill, the two smallest. Historically, military training centers have been associated with seasonal respiratory outbreaks during the first few weeks of training and have been ideal populations for FRI and influenza surveillance (Faix, 2006). The population is well-defined, historic data are available, FRI cases are known and accessible, and influenza vaccination is universal.

Surveillance is population-based. FRI incidence is pathogen-specific. NRDL hires, trains, and supervises the research assistant responsible for surveillance at each site. Throat swab samples are collected from trainees with an oral temperature greater than 38°C and a cough or sore throat, or from any case of provider-diagnosed pneumonia. Case data are recorded. The research assistant at each site ships frozen samples to NRDL at pre-arranged frequencies or weekly during influenza season. As in all NRDL surveillance activities, samples are first tested in the molecular biology laboratory before being passed to cell culture.

Additional specimens have increased confidence in the estimates of how effective influenza vaccine has been in preventing laboratory-confirmed influenza (Russell et al., 2005). This very imaginative use of the FRI provides a valuable rapid assessment of vaccine effectiveness—and thus the degree of correlation of the vaccine in use and the prevalent influenza strain early in the influenza season. The NRDL found that the overall vaccine effectiveness in 2006-2007 for the study population was 90 percent.

FRI surveillance data from the eight military training sites are a resource representing each section of the country and each branch of the military. Standard surveillance methodologies, on-site NRDL staff, and sample testing in a single laboratory (NRDL) make it possible to compare disease burdens at each site. Evaluation of factors contributing to site-specific FRI rates may lead to DoD-wide improvements in the trainee health environment.

Conclusions

The site-specific measurements of the effectiveness of influenza vaccine generated each season by NRDL are a unique national resource with important implications for annual national and international vaccine selection. Annual virus-effectiveness comparisons of live and inactivated vaccines could provide valuable information on the level of protection provided by each in the event of a major antigenic drift. In addition, factors contributing to trends or changes in site-specific FRI rates may be of particular importance in developing strategies for reducing or diminishing the frequency of cases of FRI among trainees. Annual site-specific influenza virus-effectiveness data (differentiated by live and inactivated) made available by NRDL could also make a larger DoD contribution at the annual February meeting of the Food and Drug Administration influenza vaccine strain selection subcommittee.

RECOMMENDATION 8-1. NRDL should investigate factors contributing to the ability or inability of the eight military training sites to meet maximum FRI surveillance targets as well as continue to explore methods to validate the reliability of vaccine-effectiveness data, which are available from no other populations on a consistent basis.

Shipboard FRI Surveillance

Shipboard surveillance was initiated in 2002. Navy personnel make port calls throughout the world in places where influenza or other respiratory pathogens may emerge. Exposures to respiratory diseases at ports of call greatly enhance worldwide surveillance and could provide early documentation of emerging pathogens. The shipboard populations, whether in port or deployed, represent well-immunized populations (greater than 90 percent immunized for influenza). Influenza outbreaks among these sentinel populations would be indicative of an influenza strain or strains for which the current vaccine provides reduced or no protection. Representative strains may be made available to U.S. and World Health Organization laboratories more quickly through these populations than through individual countries.

FRI shipboard surveillance represents a population of approximately 50,000 personnel aboard ships of the Third Fleet (seven ships) in San Diego, the Second Fleet (six ships) based in Virginia, and the Seventh Fleet (three ships) based in Japan (Faix, 2006). The basic concept is that FRI throat samples are collected and frozen in liquid nitrogen or –70°C freezers and shipped to NRDL for laboratory diagnosis upon return to port. If more rapid testing is warranted, arrangements are made to transport samples to NRDL as soon as possible. In addition to influenza surveillance, the findings would help define the relative importance of pathogens responsible for FRI, describe shipboard transmission, lead to appropriate preventive measures, and help maintain ship readiness.

The fleet has requested that NRDL assist in expanding shipboard diagnostic capability, both with polymerase chain reaction (PCR) technology and new, validated rapid tests, particularly for avian influenza. Achieving this goal presents numerous challenges, including the competency levels of technical staff on board ship, competition from other duties, the need to train staff, staff turnover, available laboratory space, and, especially, access to simple and reliable technology. NRDL continues to evaluate promising technology, with considerable attention given to quality assurance. The Centers for Disease Control and Prevention (CDC) Laboratory Response Network (LRN) H5 test is a possible candidate.

Complicating shipboard surveillance—and to a lesser extent recruit surveillance—is the potential interpretation that such programs represent research and thus require informed consent. As the number of fleet commands, ship commanders, and institutional review boards increases, completing the protocol review and informed-consent requirements become increasingly more time consuming. Longer and more complicated consent forms are a disincentive to both staff and patient for sample collection and enrollment in FRI surveillance.

Conclusions

Shipboard FRI surveillance is a valuable augmentation to global influenza surveillance efforts. The IOM committee commends NRDL staff on their commitment and their caution in responding to the requests of the command to introduce rapid-testing capability on ship for avian influenza. NRDL's heavy investment into quality control for the program is consistent with the recognized challenges of operating complex equipment and interpreting results in the shipboard environment.

RECOMMENDATION 8-2. The services should explore interpretation of the syndromic surveillance mandate to include laboratory diagnostic testing of clinically ill subjects in order to facilitate crucial febrile respiratory illness and other infectious disease surveillance in military populations.

California-Mexico Border FRI Surveillance

Surveillance among the cross-border civilian population began in 2004 as a collaborative effort with the CDC, the San Ysidro Health Center (San Diego Co.), and Clinicas de Salud del Pueblo, Calexico (Imperial Co.) (Faix, 2006). The project is funded through CDC. The clinic population, many of whom are largely unimmunized against influenza, includes people of different age groups with a variety of respiratory pathogens. NRDL tests all samples for influenza A and adenoviruses with PCR and tests for all other agents with viral culture and bacteriology techniques. These samples provide a valuable resource for evaluating promising rapid-test systems. Simultaneous evaluation of the commercially available point-of-collection influenza test in this population proved that the performance of that test was suboptimal (Faix, 2006).

Conclusions

NRDL's collaboration in this border surveillance program is valuable for NRDL and for the region. Its participation enhances the collaborative relationship with CDC and local agencies, makes possible surveillance in a binational population that may have interaction with the large number of military in the area, and provides a high yield of beneficial samples at low cost.

Expanded Surveillance Capacity

NRDL is collaborating with the U.S. Naval Hospital in Yokosuka, Japan, to establish a Pacific Rim surveillance hub (NHRC, 2006a). The rationale for establishing this hub stems from the number of shipboard influenza clusters that have occurred after port stops in the Pacific Rim area, the presence of avian influenza in the area, and the absence of capacity in the region for sample collection, testing, and shipment. Permission to proceed has been granted by the Seventh Fleet command, the hospital, and the hospital laboratory director. Office and laboratory space has been made available in the hospital, a LightCycler has been purchased, and a research assistant has been hired to organize the activity. A search for a qualified study coordinator is underway. NRDL is also assisting the Air Force Institute for Operational Health (AFIOH) in increasing sample collection and processing at its five base sentinel sites in Japan and is interfacing with Seventh Fleet preventive medicine personnel to provide FRI surveillance for upcoming deployment and exercises.

Conclusions

Establishment of the Pacific Rim surveillance hub is a logical extension of current NRDL surveillance activities. NRDL personnel on site will greatly strengthen surveillance in the area.

LABORATORY

The NRDL currently has a fully operational biosafety level 2 (BSL-2) influenza diagnostic laboratory, and a BSL-3E laboratory is under construction (NHRC, 2006a). Virus detection, identification, and sub-typing are performed in the molecular biology laboratory (PCR, subtyping, and gene sequencing) and followed by culture of positive samples and selected negatives in the virology division (culture, identification via direct or indirect immunofluorescence, and hemagglutination inhibition serotyping) of the microbiology laboratory.

The supplemental funding for avian influenza/pandemic influenza (AI/PI) has been allocated to expanding or enhancing physical structure and laboratory capacity in several important ways. First, it has been used to increase the laboratory surge capacity, allowing for the collection of a greater number of specimens than was previously possible. This has been accomplished through the use of reverse transcriptase PCR (RT-PCR) screening of samples in a high throughput format. Currently, these samples are handled in the BSL-2 facilities.

Second, a BSL-3E facility is under construction that will, when it is completed, enhance the capabilities of the DoD in the Pacific Rim region to safely manage human pathogens of high consequence. BSL-3E facilities staffed and equipped to work with influenza A viruses of high consequence are in short supply in California. Additionally, in the Pacific Rim region, there are no other existing DoD BSL-3E facilities. The BSL-3E facility will add new challenges that may not yet have been fully anticipated. The regulatory requirements for containment facilities are shifting and will continue to change in the future. Funding for the annual maintenance and required upgrades of the BSL-3E facility is critical to maintain its functional use, and a functioning facility is a critical need for the DoD-GEIS program.

Third, personnel who add substantial expertise to the laboratory have been hired. These individuals have been able to explore cutting-edge biotechnology that can increase capacity and improve data quality and the rapid identification of the viruses detected.

Fourth, laboratories have been added in the surveillance network, including shipboard efforts and one overseas hospital (Yokosuka).

Finally, additional freezers have been purchased so that samples can be archived appropriately.

With a median time of seven days, cell culture methods for influenza A and B viruses seem to be overly time-consuming. The NHRC team has sought to overcome this time lag by directly sequencing positive samples, but challenges remain.

Quality control is a significant priority at NHRC. There are a number of checks that have been instituted internally to monitor the validity of findings, in addition to those checks prescribed by CAP and CLIP. Additionally, a full-time position has been added to oversee issues of quality assurance.

Conclusions

The NHRC team has thought through the testing and reporting of each sample that is received. Although the completeness of these planning efforts has led to the laboratories, staff, and management being highly effective in achieving the goals of the current surveillance efforts as well as in anticipating future needs, the time-consuming cell culture methods for influenza A and B viruses are a challenge that can and should be overcome.

RESPONSE CAPACITY

In terms of the three pillars of the National Strategy for Pandemic Influenza—preparedness and communication, surveillance and detection, and response and containment—NRDL interprets its mandate as the second. Supplemental 2006 funding greatly enhanced capacity for influenza surveillance and detection. Laboratory surge capacity has been increased, high-capacity cutting-edge diagnostics have been introduced, the Pacific Rim surveillance hub has been established, shipboard surveillance has been expanded, and a BSL-3E laboratory is under construction. Rigorous validation tests are under way on multiple novel procedures to identify influenza strains with high strain-specific sensitivity using original specimens.

Outbreak Response

NHRC is well positioned to assist in the response to infectious disease outbreaks in the San Diego area as well as in relevant military personnel populations. The following are a few outbreaks in which NHRC contributed to the response and investigation:

- NHRC identified an early season cluster of influenza A at Marine Corps Recruit Depot (MCRD) San Diego in August 2006. Laboratory staff quickly determined that an H1N1 strain was responsible and that none of the cases had been vaccinated. Information was immediately shared with MCRD San Diego, GEIS headquarters, CDC, and local public heath officials. FRI surveillance was intensified at this site for several weeks until it was determined that transmission had ceased. Training operations at the base were allowed to continue uninterrupted, in large part due to the epidemiological data provided by NHRC.
- Four separate outbreaks of Group A streptococcal illness among basic trainees occurred during fiscal year 2006, and NHRC provided laboratory and epidemiological support for all. In all four outbreaks, *emm* type 5 *Streptococcus pyogenes* was the predominant subtype isolated.
- An outbreak of severe pneumonia that required hospitalization of some patients occurred among Navy SEAL trainees in March 2006. NHRC was notified and worked with the Navy Environmental and Preventive Medicine Unit No. 5 to obtain and test specimens from the outbreak; *Streptococcus pneumoniae* (type 31) was identified as the etiologic agent, and appropriate treatment and prophylaxis were initiated.
- NHRC also provided laboratory support for 11 fatal or severe respiratory illness cases during fiscal year 2006. Most of these were referred through the mortality surveillance program at the Armed Forces Institute of Pathology (AFIP). Key findings included determination that *emm* type 5 *Streptococcus pyogenes* was isolated in two fatal cases among active-duty service members in Texas and that *Streptococcus pneumoniae* was associated with another fatal case.
- NHRC provided weekly updates that included influenza and FRI rate data to surveillance partners throughout the year.
- NHRC provided rapid laboratory confirmation of adenoviral etiology during FRI rate spikes that were identified by the FRI surveillance

program. These spikes occurred at six of eight camps under surveillance during fiscal year 2006.

Surge Capacity

NRDL performs routine molecular screening on approximately 168 samples per week. Samples are extracted in a 96-well format (two plates) that includes a total of 12 internally placed positive and negative controls per plate (NHRC, 2007) (see Table 8-1).

NRDL would initially be able to alter its current testing algorithm to test for only influenza A first and then H5 if positive. This would allow the screening of an additional 504 samples per week, for a total of 672 samples per week (NHRC, 2007). NRDL does stock supplies, but only sufficient quantities for a defined "high throughput" period of operation (see below). Further refinement of the screening process, targeting only the gene required to rule in or out the strain of interest, would allow NRDL to more than double the altered algorithm and total throughput to approximately 1,548 samples. This would require reassignment of some staff to focus on these efforts (NHRC, 2007).

In an emergency situation, NRDL could transition into a 24-hour operation, doubling again the number of samples processed. The best estimates of NRDL short-term surge capability would result in a throughput of 3,528 samples per week using the lab's standard molecular capabilities (NHRC, 2007). Again, this would require reassigning staff to focus only on these activities. The limiting factor would not be the laboratory or equipment, but rather—eventually—reagents.

In order to help with a surge in sample processing and rapid identification, NRDL has advanced diagnostic compatibility that would help identify type and strain of circulating influenzas. This technology would be able to process 176 samples in a 24-hour period (NHRC, 2007). Validation efforts for the College of American Pathology certification are near completion. Although the advanced diagnostic equipment may not be able to test all

TABLE 8-1 Summary of Surge Capability at the NRDL, NHRC

Condition	PCR	T-5000	Total
Routine operation	168/week	168/week	336/week
Altered algorithm — influenza A and H5 first	672/week	440/week	1,112/week
Target only specific gene	1,548/week	440/week	1,988/week
24-hour operations	3,528/week	1,232/week	4,760/week

SOURCE: NHRC, 2007.

positive specimens during a pandemic, testing a systematic sample of positives would provide much additional information about circulating strains in much less time than traditional methods.

A potential problem with high-throughput processing is the rate at which reagents and consumables are used. In the event that pandemic influenza transmission is thought to be occurring, it is likely that routine shipping sources would slow. In preparation for any 24-hour processing scenario, NRDL is now preparing stockpiles of consumables and reagents that would allow the laboratory to maintain a 24-hour operation for one month in the event of a national emergency (NHRC, 2007). NRDL will rotate reagents with new orders when received, thus maintaining the surge capability indefinitely and without additional cost or risk of wasted reagents.

Conclusions

NRDL is a highly focused operation with well-qualified staff dedicated to its mission. This laboratory is poised to play a valuable leadership role in identifying and responding to a potential influenza pandemic.

COLLABORATION AND COORDINATION

NHRC has established a number of strategically advantageous relationships with U.S. government agencies (including those within the DoD) as well as academic and private organizations. NRDL works closely with the CDC in sharing influenza isolates and with Lawrence Livermore National Laboratory and multiple manufacturers in the evaluation of rapid diagnostic tests for installation and field (shipboard) applications. NRDL and AFIOH collaborated on quality-control testing and in exercises designed to facilitate testing backup in the event one or the other laboratory was overwhelmed with influenza samples. Ties are close with training sites, fleet commands, and each of the overseas laboratories. By design there are no direct collaborations with foreign governments or international organizations; NHRC relies instead on the naval medical research units and fleet bases to provide those channels. Contacts with the U.S. Department of Agriculture are through certification for importation of animal isolates, and contacts with CDC are through importation of human samples. Additionally, NRDL collaborates with CDC and local health authorities on the cross-border project. Collaborations should be explored with local health departments and relevant university departments as well as the local veterinary community to promote and increase communication and information sharing within the region.

REFERENCES

Faix, D. 2006. *Febrile respiratory illness surveillance and research at Naval Health Research Center: Evaluating unique populations*. PowerPoint presentation at first meeting of the IOM Committee for the Assessment of DoD-GEIS, December 19, Washington, DC.

NHRC (Naval Health Research Center). 2006a. *NHRC project titles and descriptions*. (unpublished).

NHRC. 2006b. *FY06 annual summary report* (Unpublished).

NHRC. 2007. *Laboratory surge capacity*. (unpublished).

Russell K. L., Ryan M. A. , Hawksworth A., Freed N. E., Irvine M., Daum L.T. 2005. Effectiveness of the 2003-2004 influenza vaccine among U.S. military basic trainees: A year of suboptimal match between vaccine and circulating strain. *Vaccine* Mar 14; 23(16):1981-1985.

LIST OF CONTACTS

DoD-GEIS NHRC Assessment: San Diego, California

Lt. Cmdr. Dennis Faix, Naval Health Research Center, San Diego, California
Julie Fuller, Naval Health Research Center, San Diego, California
Tony Hawksworth, Naval Health Research Center, San Diego, California
Marina Irvine, Naval Health Research Center, San Diego, California
Dr. Pete Kammerer, Naval Health Research Center, San Diego, California
Dr. David Metzgar, Naval Health Research Center, San Diego, California
Dr. Chris Myers, Naval Health Research Center, San Diego, California
Miguel Angel Osuna, Naval Health Research Center, San Diego, California
Cmdr. Kevin Russell, Naval Health Research Center, San Diego, California
Margaret Ryan, Naval Health Research Center, San Diego, California

SCHEDULE OF EVENTS

DoD-GEIS NHRC Assessment
San Diego, California
Participants: Dr. Carol J. Cardona
Dr. Walter R. Dowdle
Kimberly Weingarten
March 26-27, 2007

Monday, March 26, 2007

0800-0830	Breakfast
0830-0840	**Welcome remarks**
0840-0900	**Introduction to Naval Respiratory Disease Laboratory activities** Cmdr. Kevin Russell
0900-0940	**Discussion about febrile respiratory illness surveillance in U.S. military basic training centers** Tony Hawksworth
0940-1010	**Discussion about global naval shipboard surveillance** Cmdr. Kevin Russell
1040-1040	**Discussion about Pacific Rim surveillance hub** Dr. Peter Kammerer
1100-1100	Break

1100-1130	**Discussion about surveillance in the United States-Mexico border region** Tony Hawksworth
1200-1200	**Discussion on DoD support** Lt. Cmdr. Dennis Faix
1200-1330	Lunch
1330-1430	**Tour of U.S. Navy ship**
1500-1600	**Tour of branch medical clinic at Marine Corps Recruit Depot**

Tuesday, March 27, 2007

0800-0830	Breakfast
0830-0850	**Welcome remarks and introduction to MRDL research projects** Cmdr. Kevin Russell
0850-0920	**Discussion about laboratory testing** Miguel Angel Osuna
0920-1000	**Discussion about the sequencing of 100 percent of influenza isolates** Dr. Chris Myers
1000-1020	Break
1020-1100	**Discussion about the influenza differentiation between wild type and vaccine (FluMist©)** Dr. Dave Metzgar
1100-1130	**Evaluations of advanced diagnostic platforms** Cmdr. Kevin Russell
1130-1200	**Discussion about expanding capabilities through technology-transfer training or an advanced diagnostic laboratory** Lt. Cmdr. Dennis Faix
1200-1230	**Discussion about BSL-3E laboratory** Julie Fuller
1330-1330	Lunch
1500-1500	**Tour of NRDL facilities**
1600-1600	**Final discussion, farewells**
1600-	Departure

9

Air Force Institute for Operational Health San Antonio Avian and Pandemic Influenza Activities

The U.S. Air Force began its global influenza surveillance of U.S. military forces and their families in 1976 under Project Gargle (AFIOH, 2006b). Through this program the Air Force systematically collected febrile respiratory illness (FRI) specimens from clinics and hospitals worldwide. In 1997 these efforts were expanded with the development by the Department of Defense (DoD) of the Global Laboratory-Based Influenza Surveillance Program. At the same time, the Office of the Assistant Secretary of Defense for Health Affairs designated the Surgeon General of the Air Force as the executive agent for DoD influenza surveillance (Bailey, 1999). This policy expanded influenza surveillance and promoted a more DoD-wide approach, including sentinel site surveillance of U.S. military personnel and DoD beneficiaries, DoD global medical research facilities, and non-U.S. military forces.

The organization of the DoD Global Emerging Infections Surveillance and Response System (DoD-GEIS) created a DoD-wide global influenza surveillance network that encompassed and expanded the Air Force's Project Gargle and the Navy's population-based surveillance of recruits. A DoD policy, *Health Affairs Policy Memo 99-081*, was signed, and the Air Force Surgeon General was appointed as the executive agent of the new DoD Global Laboratory-Based Influenza Surveillance Program, with management responsibility given to the Air Force Institute for Operational Health (AFIOH) (AFIOH, 2006b). The AFIOH core program for influenza surveillance is guided by both the *Health Affairs Policy Memo 99-081* and the *Department of Defense Implementation Plan for Pandemic In-*

fluenza. DoD-GEIS provided funding, programmatic support, and professional guidance to the Air Force in administering this new program, which then became two-pronged (AFIOH, 2006b, DoD, 2006). One prong was surveillance among U.S. military personnel and DoD medical beneficiaries; the second was surveillance in civilian populations in areas of the world where DoD units were located and which were suited to surveillance and to the providing of support to host country populations and allied countries. AFIOH also contributes to the Vaccines and Related Biological Products Advisory Committee (VRBPAC) of the U.S. Food and Drug Administration (FDA) and the Armed Forces Epidemiological Board now known as the Defense Health Board.

A site visit team of the Institute of Medicine (IOM) Committee for the Assessment of DoD-GEIS Influenza Surveillance and Response Programs visited AFIOH on March 28-29, 2007.[1] A list of the people met and interviewed and the itinerary followed can be found at the end of this chapter.

MANAGEMENT AND PLANNING

While the majority of the avian influenza/pandemic influenza (AI/PI) supplemental funding has been allocated to personnel costs, it does not appear that personnel dedicated to assure quality were added as each section was expanded. The AFIOH laboratory has a rigorous quality-assurance program associated with its College of American Pathologists (CAP) and Clinical Laboratory Improvement Program (CLIP) accreditations. However, the lack of technical expertise in particular areas has limited the effectiveness and sustainability of AFIOH's expanded AI/PI surveillance and detection program.

AFIOH has spent a significant portion of the AI/PI supplemental funds on one-time-only expenditures, and it expects that the increase in capacity, particularly in molecular biology, data management, and added surveillance sites, can be maintained in the future with an annual funding level of approximately equal to one-third of the $4.1 million AFIOH received.

The AFIOH program is expecting a move to Wright-Patterson Air Force Base in Dayton, Ohio, by 2011, and personnel involved in the influenza program are aware that this move will be a challenge for their program. The issues that they expect include retaining personnel in San Antonio until the site closes, side-by-side operations for some period of time, the potential need to rebuild the program in Dayton, and the reluctance to make neces-

[1]Prior to the committee's visit to AFIOH, the laboratory staff provided the committee with detailed background information on AFIOH and the pandemic/avian influenza activities it was supporting. These materials were used in the writing of this chapter and are available from the IOM in the Public Access File.

sary improvements in the current building or campus. The move and its impact are expected to be a major challenge, and the team at AFIOH is well into planning how to overcome any issues that may arise.

Staffing

The Air Force Institute for Operational Health (AFIOH) has two divisions that deal with the surveillance program for viral and bacterial agents. Staff in these divisions often split their time between the influenza program and other AFIOH research activities. One division focuses on the epidemiology of different agents and employs about 24 people. The second division, dealing with laboratory identification, has about 95 people, of whom 23 are responsible for the packing and receiving of samples. Five employees are responsible for customer service, which involves interacting with other laboratories both nationally and internationally. The committee was told that 1.4 million samples are handled annually.

The DoD-GEIS-driven program for influenza includes sentinel site surveillance among U.S. military personnel and DoD beneficiaries, at DoD global medical research facilities, and among non-U.S. military forces. In addition, influenza surveillance is done on several civilian populations around the world where DoD units are located and local support is conducive to such activities. A subset of the above AFIOH staff (33 people in total) is working on influenza-related activities. Many of these 33 people are working on multiple projects, and seven represent AFIOH leadership overseeing all of the projects at the laboratory. Two-thirds (about 22 employees) are part of the base funding derived from DoD-GEIS funds. Nine or ten people are employed through the DoD-GEIS supplemental program, which is aimed at dealing with the threat posed by a new influenza pandemic. AFIOH is thus charged with expanding the capabilities to do high-throughput screening for influenza and to identify increased disease activity, allowing for an adequate and timely response to a pandemic. Currently, there are 65 sites in 40 countries from which samples can be obtained. The isolation frequency (25 percent) of influenza A and B virus isolates is high and speaks to an effective staff capable in classical isolation methodologies.

However, the IOM committee found the capability of staff in modern molecular techniques to be less effective. The lack of cutting edge technical expertise in this area has limited the effectiveness, sustainability, and potential of AFIOH's expanded AI/PI surveillance and detection program. In early 2007, there were major staffing problems in the molecular biology section. The departure of key molecular biology personnel appears to have deprived the entire section of much-needed expertise. Unfortunately, the AFIOH leadership may not be aware that the remaining staff is not up to date in molecular biologic techniques. The committee felt that this lack of expertise, in combination with the associated challenges identifying and addressing issues of quality in the molecular biology program, despite having standard AFIOH quality assurance protocols on hand, threaten the effectiveness and limit the potential of the section's influenza surveillance activities.

The epidemiology staff is charged with tracking the effectiveness of influenza vaccination and the epidemiological pattern of individuals participating in the DoD-GEIS influenza surveillance program. It is not clear that the present staff has the experience and the determination to collect the necessary raw data and then to provide compelling epidemiological assessments. Specifically, both the laboratory staff and the epidemiology staff need strengthening to reliably and confidently find new pandemic strains or to identify unusual epidemiological situations. The laboratory does not aggressively test for non-H1 and non-H3 influenza virus strains and does not proactively solicit samples for timely analysis. We were told that samples from Peru are frequently six months old. The epidemiological surveillance appears to be passive rather than proactive and lags behind in applying modern algorithms.

Technology and Information Management

Under the fiscal year 2006 AI/PI supplemental funding, three information management/information technology (IM/IT) analysts are being supported to add and improve capabilities in three principal areas. First, a computer-based sample labeling and tracking system is being put into place to replace the time-consuming and error-prone manual procedures currently used. Second, geographic mapping software is being acquired to provide all stakeholders with interactive access to influenza-like illness (ILI) data from medical treatment facilities. (Even without this capability, a great deal of further analysis should be done with this data; for instance, seeking out trends by geographic region or demographic group, rather than just the current breakdown by military service branch.) Finally, a large centralized database is being set up to collect DoD encounter data: visits, prescriptions, etc. by all active and retired military personnel and their dependents, both at DoD medical treatment facilities and non-DoD facilities. This effort appears to be still in the planning stages, and we would strongly encourage a close coordination with other related DoD-wide efforts, such as the Medical Data Access Real-Time framework, which is used to mine composite health care system data from DoD medical treatment facilities and is coordinated by the Office of the Secretary of Defense Clinical Information Technology Program Office.

Data analysis efforts at AFIOH primarily involve the collection, analysis, and reporting of ILI activity at DoD military treatment facilities worldwide. Standard Ambulatory Data Registry data is collected on a weekly basis from Air Force sites and on a monthly basis for other service branches. Any site experiencing an increase in respiratory patient visits (defined as more than two standard deviations above the mean) is notified and asked to provide specimen samples. Graphs showing overall ILI activity among each service branch are included in the weekly Influenza Surveillance Update published by AFIOH. In addition, DoD-wide respiratory disease laboratory data gathered through the composite health care system is collected and uploaded to the Centers for Disease Control and Prevention (CDC) on a weekly basis.

The ILI tracking program is systematically connected with a trigger to communicate unusual occurrences of ILI back to participating sites. These communications are critical and allow for real-time responses to clusters of illness as they occur.

The AFIOH team has shared its accumulated experience and expertise in shipping and receiving with its sentinel sites and the public in general. This is done through an extensive description of packing protocols that is provided in writing, upon request, and is fully available on the internet. Similarly, communications about how to collect nasal washes are excellent.

Conclusions

Given the demonstrated importance of the AFIOH to the U.S. and WHO programs for identifying influenza vaccine strains, it must be staffed and led by individuals with the best reputations in public health laboratory virology and respiratory disease epidemiology. The molecular biology capacity of AFIOH cannot be maintained in light of the current lack of expertise in personnel in the molecular biology section and a lack of expertise in molecular biology among the leadership. The lack of expertise hinders this group from fully utilizing the resources at its disposal, and it must be addressed in order to make this program sustainable. Permanent expertise in molecular biology and data management is critical, but short-term advisors might be helpful in solving immediate problems. The lack of molecular biology expertise at AFIOH will prevent the accurate presentation of this data to stakeholders such as VRBPAC. This lack of expertise has and will continue to affect the effective functioning of AFIOH in communications.

RECOMMENDATION 9-1. AFIOH's influenza program should employ a strong doctoral-level molecular biologist with demonstrated technical and leadership skills. These should include a strong background in laboratory quality control methods. The program staff should be

well-versed in the data analytic approaches desired by the FDA influenza vaccine committee. The laboratory should regularly obtain technical guidance from appropriate sources (e.g., CDC, FDA, academia, and GEIS headquarters) to ensure that it is using state-of-the-art methods and is targeting appropriate specimen sources.

SURVEILLANCE

The program at AFIOH provides national and international respiratory disease data from DoD beneficiaries within the U.S. Air Force, Army, Navy, and Coast Guard. Allied nations in areas cooperating with the DoD overseas medical research facilities are also collaborating partners. Surveillance is conducted under three areas at AFIOH. The first is surveillance for influenza-like illness (ILI); the second surveillance effort involves the testing of samples from enrolled sentinel sites; and the third entails the testing of clinical samples arriving from all over the world for a variety of illness complaints (AFIOH, 2007b).

The ILI surveillance program collects clinical data on the number of ILI cases occurring at enrolled surveillance sites. This effort has resulted in near real-time collection of clinical cases meeting the DoD ILI definition across the services. These data are compiled by the epidemiology team at AFIOH, and any sites experiencing an incidence of ILI two standard deviations above the average are contacted by AFIOH.

The flagship surveillance program for AFIOH is the former Project Gargle (started in 1976), now known simply as sentinel site surveillance. Currently, there are 56 sentinel sites in 34 countries, the majority of which are military and DoD research sites or hospitals overseas (see Figure 9.1) (AFIOH, 2007b).

New sites are under consideration for addition. Factors considered in the selection of a sentinel site are the potential for emergence of new strains of influenza virus, the potential for importation of new strains, the impact of an outbreak or novel influenza virus on military operations, and whether an area has high troop concentrations and highly mobile or rapid-response units. Sentinel sites are required to institute an active influenza surveillance and identification program. They submit weekly specimens collected from patients meeting the criteria for influenza-like illness (ILI) (i.e., fever of more than 38°C and cough or sore throat) along with a completed influenza surveillance questionnaire to provide an epidemiological profile (AFIOH, 2006a). Passive surveillance is performed at non-sentinel sites; the patients from whom respiratory specimens are collected at those sites do not necessarily meet ILI criteria (i.e., they are not always clinical respiratory diagnostic specimens). AFIOH provides sentinel sites with a program brochure describing the program, an educational presentation, staff-specific

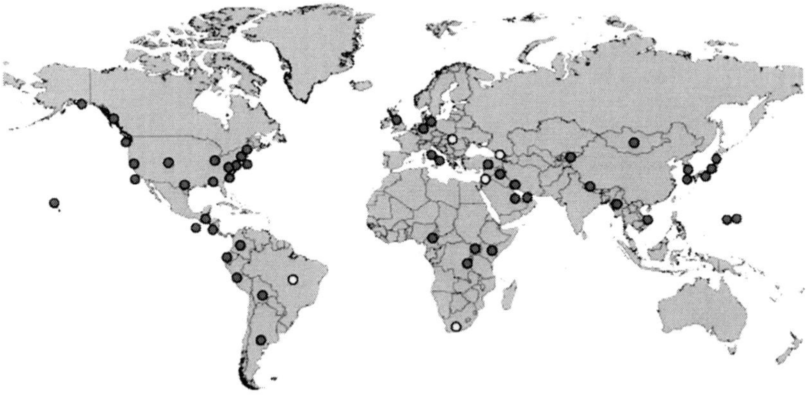

FIGURE 9-1 AFIOH sentinel surveillance sites and activities, present and future, 2006-2007.
SOURCE: Neville, 2006.

educational pamphlets, a guidance sheet, influenza surveillance questionnaires, and specimen collection kits.

Sites are requested to collect six to ten viral culture specimens per week along with case data from patients meeting the ILI case definition. Specimens are collected as throat or nasopharyngeal swabs or nasal wash using viral transport medium (MicroTest M4-RT [Remel, Lenexa, KS]). Specimens collected from U.S. locations are refrigerated, shipped on gel packs, and received within three to four shipping days. All other specimens are frozen at -70°C and shipped on dry ice by a commercial carrier. Upon arrival, specimens are processed in a biosafety level 2 (BSL-2) laboratory (BSL-3 is available) and cultured for isolation of influenza A, influenza B, adenovirus, parainfluenza virus 1, 2, and 3, enterovirus, respiratory syncytial virus, and herpes simplex virus using rhesus monkey K cells. Specimens are cultured for up to 10 days before negative results are reported. All original samples are maintained in the event that they are needed to supply a vaccine seed virus. Only original sample material for growth in eggs is acceptable for vaccine production. All influenza isolates collected from locations outside the United States and isolates of interest from the United States are subtyped using hemagglutination-inhibition (HI) or reverse transcriptase polymerase chain reaction (RT-PCR) procedures. A sample of these isolates undergoes molecular sequencing at AFIOH to identify significant amino acid changes. Select isolates and all sequence data are sent to the CDC for further subtyping and antigenic characterization for detection of variance from the vaccine component strains. All fiscal year 2006 AFIOH influenza surveillance data, which are to include 120 isolates and 101 original samples, have been shared with CDC and the World Health Organization (WHO).

The AI/PI supplemental funding has been used specifically to increase laboratory staffing to test additional incoming samples and to provide shipping supplies and updated educational materials on how to properly ship samples.

The AFIOH laboratory is a busy clinical laboratory. Any U.S. military site can submit clinical respiratory specimens to AFIOH. Twenty-three non-sentinel sites have been tested since October 2006 after submitting samples to AFIOH for evaluation and were also included in influenza A and B surveillance. The patients tested in this program do not necessarily meet the DoD case definition for ILI.

Conclusions

AFIOH's efforts to pull together surveillance data from all of the services have been hampered by a lack of cooperation and the inability to collect standardized data. These data are valuable for tracking disease clusters and should be analyzed in the largest aggregate group that is possible. The designated reporting agency for surveillance would be able to coordinate information more effectively and efficiently if the data from all participants were received in a timely and fully analyzable manner. This relates to Recommendation 10.1.

LABORATORY

AFIOH is the central laboratory for the DoD influenza program. It serves as both a clinical and a public health laboratory, generating both active and passive surveillance data. AFIOH occupies a large laboratory building at Brooks City Base, located just south of San Antonio, Tex. The space was built in the 1960s and houses numerous BSL-2 laboratories, a single BSL-3 suite, and office spaces, which are not biohazard-handling spaces. Access to the laboratory space is generally restricted by control of the front door of the building. Additionally, the designated Laboratory Response Network (LRN) space is controlled and limited to selected employees (14 people total) as is access to the 240-square-foot BSL-3 space in the building (four people total). Other rooms in the building that are designated BSL-2 spaces are identified with prominent biohazard signs.

The molecular biology section is currently being remodeled to more closely approximate a useful configuration for the laboratory. At the present time, traffic flow, separation of the steps in the processing of samples, and the essential controls needed to prevent and detect contamination are all lacking. The molecular biology section is housed in two contiguous rooms linked by two doors. Samples from the virology section arrive in the laboratory for testing in a fully infectious state. They are inactivated, processed for RT-PCR, and tested (RT-PCR screening, subtyping, and sequencing) in these two rooms. All extracted RNA and any archived products are kept in two ultra-low-temperature freezers in the molecular biology laboratory suite. It is unclear how and where any positive controls for molecular biology tests are stored and handled, including any that are on site for the detection of novel HA and NA subtypes.

The volume of incoming packages, with approximately 1.4 million samples arriving annually from multiple laboratories and surveillance sites around the world, presents a major space issue for the laboratory (AFIOH, 2006b). Among the incoming samples are approximately 1,600 submitted annually for influenza A and B detection. Samples for influenza A and B testing flow from the designated shipping and receiving areas to the virology laboratory, where they are inoculated onto cultures. The shipping and receiving management is outstanding in this laboratory.

Classical virological methods are used for the initial detection of influenza A viruses in clinical samples. These methods include dual inoculation of shell vials and culture tubes. Viruses are cultured for 24 to 48 hours and then detected with IFA techniques. The isolation rates achieved for the laboratory (approximately 40 percent) would indicate that the staff and the methods used are highly effective.

The space and equipment dedicated to the ultra-low-temperature storage of samples and viruses for normal storage and archiving is not sufficient for the storage of more than one year's sample volume. Additionally, there is currently no liquid nitrogen storage in the virology laboratory, which limits long-term storage of cells.

The current methods for labeling tubes and tracking samples are inadequate for the sample volume coming into this laboratory and may introduce error into the system. Currently, tube inserts are labeled by hand and a preprinted label is attached to the tube. Two tubes are labeled and a single sample divided between them. These tubes are then placed into cardboard boxes and then into ultra-low-temperature freezers.

Conclusions

The AFIOH laboratory does well with virus isolation, which is now done in only a few places. This is a valuable service offered by AFIOH and should be supported. However, it is critical that the laboratory work with partners to further maximize the use of valuable samples collected by the DoD influenza program (both original patient samples and virus samples).

There are a variety of organizations which may be able to assist in this, such as the National Institutes of Health (NIH).

There is inadequate attention paid to preventing and controlling contamination, particularly in the molecular biology section. The potential for contamination was a major concern of the committee, and the refitting that is currently underway will not address this problem.

RECOMMENDATION 9-2. **In order to minimize potential for contamination in the molecular biology section and to improve the data generated by this section, AFIOH should seek expertise in molecular biology techniques and their implementation in a diagnostic laboratory setting.**

While the sample flow from different international sites appears to be adequate, the present staff has not taken full advantage of modern diagnostic techniques. For example, in the AFIOH weekly influenza surveillance report of March 18-24, 2007, it is suggested that "over 90 percent of the influenza isolates have been molecularly sequenced." In fact, only the hemagglutinin genes had been sequenced (not the entire viral genome) and most likely only the HA1 portion. Furthermore, state-of-the-art multiplex technologies have not been installed at AFIOH, while some collaborating laboratories overseas (and also domestically) effectively use such techniques in their surveillance efforts.

RECOMMENDATION 9-3. **AFIOH should consider the expansion of its laboratory capacity to include multi-tasking diagnostic equipment for respiratory diseases.**

The archival storage of original sample material and virus isolates, an important resource coming from this laboratory, is inadequate. The sample labeling system could easily introduce error, as could the lack of an orderly data management system. The equipment needed for sustaining appropriate archived samples, both from the virology and molecular biology sections, is not sufficient to satisfy anticipated future needs.

RECOMMENDATION 9-4. **AFIOH should create a sustainable and useful archive of the original patient sample and virus isolate materials in this laboratory to ensure that this national resource can be used to fulfill the missions of the DoD-GEIS AI/PI program.**

AFIOH's use of the surveillance and sequencing data is less effective than its surveillance and specimen collection system. Collaborations with other U.S. government and scientific entities could maximize the shared knowledge resulting from the lab's surveillance activities. For example, rigorous rules should be made as to when and how data are shared with the public as well as with other organizations, such as the NIH and Los Alamos National Laboratory (LANL). The NIH has a major sequencing program of influenza virus isolates, and LANL also has a program and superb expertise for analyzing influenza virus sequence data. Both NIH and LANL have exceptional computational biologists trained in the analysis of evolutionary changes of influenza viruses.

RECOMMENDATION 9-5. AFIOH should continue collaborate with both the National Institutes of Health and Los Alamos National Laboratory and provide sequencing data and samples when appropriate.

AFIOH would also benefit from working with cutting-edge academic collaborators who could be helpful in identifying agents present in samples that have eluded identification by in-house people. For example, the Ganem and deRisi laboratories at University of California, San Francisco (UCSF) and the Lipkin laboratory at Columbia University have developed methodologies for the identification of respiratory agents. Such techniques may allow the identification of agents responsible for mixed infections and possibly result in the identification of new agents responsible for respiratory infections. Finally, AFIOH is encouraged to share reagents with other interested parties. Such sharing should occur with minimal bureaucratic interference and may be facilitated by asking for nominal fees to offset costs for preparing and shipping reagents and materials. Alternatively, agreements similar to cooperative research and development agreements could be initiated with appropriate parties interested in collaborations.

RECOMMENDATION 9-6. AFIOH should seek out cutting-edge academic collaborators in order to expand the methodologies available to identify agents responsible for mixed infections, which could possibly result in the identification of new agents responsible for respiratory infections.

RESPONSE CAPACITY

In the six months since October 1, 2006, only 1,613 samples were processed, resulting in the laboratory isolation of 414 influenza viruses. The relatively low number of processed isolates over a period of six months should allow for a considerable surge capacity should there be need for it. The AFIOH virology laboratory has a documented (February 2007) surge plan to address the increased workload for either unusually severe seasonal influenza or the potential emergence of a human pandemic strain. The two

TABLE 9-1 Summary AFIOH Surge Capacity

	8 Hours a Day, 5 Days a Week	24 Hours a Day, 7 Days a Week
Traditional RT-PCR	1,300 samples/week	5,000 samples/week
Traditional RT-PCR (1 gene target)	2,600 samples/week	11,000 samples/week
H5 LRN assay	1,500 samples/week	6,000 samples/week

SOURCE: AFIOH, 2007a.

pillars of this plan are the stockpiling of approximately 500 frozen R-Mix ReadyCells, which are regularly tested and have been validated to detect influenza in 24 to 48 hours, and the cross-training of *all* medical laboratory AFIOH personnel to assist in nasal wash specimen handling, screening, sub-typing, and sequencing. It is stated that this plan will increase the sample throughput threefold, from the present capacity of 300 specimens per day screened with RT-PCR up to 900 specimens per day. It is not clear whether the subtyping or sequencing capacities (100 and 40 specimens per day, respectively) will increase by similar factors.

Surge Capacity

Under routine conditions, the AFIOH/SDEM Molecular Diagnostics Laboratory is capable of performing molecular screening on 1,300 samples per week (see Table 9-1). AFIOH would perform the FDA-approved LRN Assay for H5 with the capacity to screen 1,500 samples per week (AFIOH, 2007a). Targeting only the gene required to rule in or rule out the strain of interest would allow screening of up to 2,600 samples per week.

If the lab transitioned to a 24-hours-a-day, 7-days-a-week operation, the estimated short-term surge capacity would be 11,000 samples per week (AFIOH, 2007a). This would require reassigning of staff from other departments in the laboratory to maintain operations. This large volume of samples would have a major impact on the department that receives and processes specimens. AFIOH has an additional stock of supplies available for a short-term surge and would work with the vendors to have additional supplies delivered overnight if needed.

Conclusions

The capacity to test additional samples is sustainable; however, with problems in such areas as sample labeling, tracking, and archiving, the increased rate of testing will result in increased errors and losses of samples (archiving issues) and thus, potentially, no real ability to increase capacity. Coherent reporting requires the input of consistent, high-quality data. In this case, data coming from a variety of institutes have been difficult to gather and, thus, have not been reported.

The currently documented surge plan contains a number of variable factors (e.g., regular vs. round-the-clock work shifts, BSL-2 or BSL-3 operations, supply inventories) which will be determined at the time that the need for increased sample rates arises, so as much preparatory work as possible is needed to smooth the final execution. In addition, given the regular turnover in personnel and the large number of opportunities for improvement revealed by previous exercises, AFIOH would benefit from periodic exercises of BSL-3 laboratory procedures similar to those carried out in December 2005.

RECOMMENDATION 9-7. AFIOH should continue to conduct periodic training exercises and dry runs in order to further develop and test the surge plan.

COLLABORATION AND COORDINATION

The AFIOH laboratory is the central laboratory for the DoD influenza program. One of the roles of AFIOH is to collaborate with many sites for the purpose of sample collection (see Box 9-1). This is done adequately and represents a strength of the program. AFIOH collects surveillance data from sentinel sites, drawing on the strategic positions of DoD overseas medical research laboratories, including the Naval Medical Research Center Detachment in Lima (collecting specimens from Argentina, Bolivia, Ecuador, Peru, and Colombia), the Armed Forces Research Institute of Medical Sciences in Bangkok (collecting specimens from local residents in Nepal, Thailand, and Vietnam), the U.S. Army Medical Research Unit-Kenya in Nairobi (collected from local residents in Burundi, Cameroon, Uganda, and Kenya), and the U.S. Army Center for Health Promotion and Preventive Medicine in Honduras (collecting specimens from local residents in El Salvador, Guatemala, Honduras, and Nicaragua) (AFIOH, 2007b). Most of the overseas medical research laboratories submitted respiratory specimens routinely throughout the 2005-2006 seasonal year.

In addition to its collaborations with the DoD overseas facilities, AFIOH provides select isolates and all sequence data to the CDC for further sub-typing and antigenic characterization for detection of variance from the vaccine component strains (AFIOH, 2007b). All fiscal year 2006 AFIOH influenza surveillance data, which is to include 120 isolates and 101 original samples, have been shared with CDC and WHO. As a result of this information sharing, a unique seed virus from one of the DoD surveillance

BOX 9-1
DoD Influenza Executive Agent Functions Identified by AFIOH

Act as the central recipient of influenza virus specimens and influenza laboratory results from all DoD medical treatment facilities that have clinical virology capability

Maintain an archive of global influenza specimens available to CDC for vaccine production considerations

Compile DoD lab-based influenza data into periodic and annual summary reports

Coordinate influenza surveillance activities with DoD-GEIS and other relevant DoD partners including conducting the annual DoD influenza surveillance coordination meeting

Coordinate with the Influenza Branch of the CDC for sharing of select isolates considered unique or otherwise warranting further characterization at CDC in the vaccine production process

Brief the FDA's Vaccine and Related Biological Products Advisory Committee (VRBPAC) and Defense Health Board (formerly AFEB) on DoD influenza surveillance results annually

Conduct outreach training and capacity-building for influenza activities

Participate in various panels, scientific and policy meetings as subject matter experts

sites forwarded to CDC by AFIOH was one of the three 2006-2007 human U.S. seasonal influenza vaccine components. The influenza B/Malaysia-like component was collected from an AFIOH sentinel site during the 2004-2005 seasonal year. During the 2005-2006 season, CDC requested AFIOH to supply influenza A/H3N2 and influenza B original samples for the upcoming Southern Hemisphere vaccine. Sixty-seven samples were provided, with 15 considered as seed candidates (AFIOH, 2007b).

In order to stay connected with the scientific community and to share findings, AFIOH staff also participate in national and international conferences, such as the meetings of the Vaccines and Related Biological Products Advisory Committee, the International Conference for Emerging Infectious Diseases, the Asia Pacific Military Medicine Conference, and the Council for State and Territorial Epidemiologists. The staff also routinely publish in scientific journals. In addition, all published sequence data are contributed to the NIH GenBank® genetic sequence database, an annotated collection of all publicly available DNA sequences (AFIOH, 2007b).

Conclusions

As the designated reporting agent in the DoD-GEIS network for influenza surveillance, AFIOH is expected to report in timely and standard ways to maximize the utility of the available data. While the newsletter produced by AFIOH is highly informative and contains excellent information, there is little or no information in the communication about data from sites outside of AFIOH.

Communication across several systems to stakeholders, clients, collaborating institutions, and the scientific community at large can be challenging. Many of the difficulties in reporting across the services are related to difficulties in the surveillance arena. There is a need to streamline and standardize reporting, which could be accomplished through a mandate to provide a standardized data feed to AFIOH. AFIOH has used communication to effectively improve surveillance efforts through improved sample quality (nasal wash instructions) and the submission of samples in a timely manner (shipping instructions). However, there is no real minimum standard for what is needed in either the collection or the reporting of data. The supplemental funding has made it more difficult to create a standard report since many sites are doing their own testing, whereas in the past most of it was done at AFIOH. This means that many laboratories and hospitals are creating their own means of reporting. The value of the surveillance data currently being collected is diminished by an inability to collect it and report it through a single entity.

The DoD influenza and respiratory disease surveillance program has evolved in recent years in response to the potential of pandemic influenza. This evolution has highlighted both the strengths and the shortcomings of the current program. In order to better reflect the current functional operating structure of DoD influenza and the respiratory disease surveillance program's chain of accountability, as well as take to advantage of AFIOH's strengths and minimize the effect of the lab's current limitations, the executive agency functions should be reexamined. (See the related recommendation in Chapter 10.)

RECOMMENDATION 9-8. In conjunction with DoD-GEIS headquarters, AFIOH should examine the current activities at AFIOH, and strategies for strengthening the AFIOH operations should be identified and supported.

REFERENCES

AFIOH (Air Force Institute for Operational Health). 2006a. *AFIOH influenza surveillance sites: DoD military-based sites* (unpublished).

AFIOH. 2006b. *The Department of Defense Global Laboratory-Based Influenza Surveillance Program: FY 2006 annual report.* San Antonio. Department of Defense

AFIOH. 2007a. *AFIOH surge capacity plan* (unpublished).

AFIOH. 2007b. *DoD-GEIS influenza surveillance and response program: AFIOH site assessment.* PowerPoint presentation given during IOM team visit to AFIOH, March 2007.

Bailey S. 1999. *Policy for DoD global, laboratory-based influenza surveillance.* Memorandum for Surgeon General of the Army, Surgeon General of the Navy, Surgeon General of the Air Force, Deputy Director for Medical Readiness, J-4, the Joint Staff. U.S. Department of Defense, Health Affairs, Washington, DC, February 3, 1999. On file with the National Academies Public Access Records Office.

DoD (Department of Defense, Office of the Assistant Secretary of Defense, and Homeland Defense). 2006. *Department of Defense implementation plan for pandemic influenza.* Washington, DC: DoD.

Neville, C. J. 2006. *Global influenza surveillance at Air Force Institute for Operational Health.* PowerPoint presentation given at first meeting of the IOM Committee for the Assessment of DoD-GEIS Influenza Surveillance and Response Programs, December 19, Washington, DC.

LIST OF CONTACTS

DoD-GEIS AFIOH Assessment: San Antonio, Texas

Paul Barnicott, Air Force Institute for Operational Health, San Antonio, Texas

Roger P. Bracio, Epidemic Outbreak Surveillance, Air Force Institute for Operational Health, San Antonio, Texas

Linda C. Canas, Epidemiological Surveillance Division, Air Force Institute for Operational Health, San Antonio, Texas

Thomas Leo Cropper, Epidemiology Services Branch, Air Force Institute for Operational Health, San Antonio, Texas

Jason Garner, Pandemic Influenza Preparedness, Air Force Institute for Operational Health, Brooks City-Base, Texas

Penny Giovanetti, 311th Human Systems Wing, Air Force Institute for Operational Health, San Antonio, Texas

Lori E. Henrichs, Epidemiological Surveillance Division, Air Force Institute for Operational Health, San Antonio, Texas

Matthew C. Johns, Pandemic Influenza Preparedness, Air Force Institute for Operational Health, Brooks City-Base, Texas

Christine Lopez, Pandemic Influenza Preparedness, Air Force Institute for Operational Health, Brooks City-Base, Texas

Samuel J.P. Livingstone, Epidemic Outbreak Surveillance Program, Lackland Air Force Base, Texas

Elizabeth Macias, Epidemiological Surveillance Division, Air Force Institute for Operational Health, San Antonio, Texas

Edwin Matos, Pandemic Influenza Preparedness, Air Force Institute for Operational Health, Brooks City-Base, Texas

Candace McCall, Risk Assessment Division, Air Force Institute for Operational Health, San Antonio, Texas

Carolyn Miller, Surveillance Directorate, Air Force Institute for Operational Health, San Antonio, Texas

James Neville, 311th Human Systems Wing, Air Force Institute for Operational Health, San Antonio, Texas

Angela Owens, Risk Assessment Division, Air Force Institute for Operational Health, San Antonio, Texas

Leslie M. Pratt, Risk Assessment Division, Air Force Institute for Operational Health, San Antonio, Texas

Ronald Rippetoe, Epidemiological Surveillance Division, Air Force Institute for Operational Health, San Antonio, Texas

Paul Sjoberg, Epidemiology Services Branch, Air Force Institute for Operational Health, San Antonio, Texas

Jose Valdez, Pandemic Influenza Preparedness, Air Force Institute for Operational Health, Brooks City-Base, Texas

Sue Worthy, Pandemic Influenza Preparedness, Air Force Institute for Operational Health, Brooks City-Base, Texas

SCHEDULE OF EVENTS

DoD-GEIS AFIOH Assessment
San Antonio, Texas
Participants: Dr. Carol Cardona
Dr. Timothy Germann
Dr. Peter Palese
Kimberly Weingarten
March 28-29, 2007

Wednesday, March 28, 2007

0800	**Arrive at Building 180 for AFIOH welcome and introductions** Met by: Col. Paul Barnicott, deputy commander, AFIOH/CV Lt. Col. Candace McCall, division chief, AFIOH/RSR Lt. Col. Paul Sjoberg, branch chief, AFIOH/RSRH Dr. Leo Cropper, Influenza Surveillance Program lead
0825	**Depart to Building 150** Escorted by: Lt. Col. Paul Sjoberg, branch chief, AFIOH/RSRH
0830-0900	**Arrive at Building 150 for 311th Human Systems Wing introductions** Met by: Col. Penny Giovanetti, deputy director, 311th HSW
0900	**Depart to Building 930**
0905-0910	**Arrive at Building 930** Met by: Col. Carolyn Miller, director, SD Lt. Col. Ronald Rippetoe, division chief, AFIOH/SDE
0910-0930	**Presentation by IOM team (introduction, goal of the visit, rules of engagement)**
0930-1040	**AFIOH Briefing—overview of program** Briefed by: Linda Canas, chief virologist, and Dr. Leo Cropper
1050-1130	**Molecular briefing** Briefed by: Dr. Elizabeth Macias, laboratory director, AFIOH
1200	Depart for lunch

1400-1430	**Data-handling efforts (Public Health Information Management System)** Briefed by: Lt Col Sjoberg/ Mr. Edwin Matos
1430-1630	**Review of the DoD-GEIS Influenza program, projects, and future plans** Interaction with AFIOH team members

Thursday, March 29, 2007

0800-1000	**Arrive at Building 180 to continue review of the DoD-GEIS influenza program, projects, and future plans** Met by: Lt, Col, Paul Sjoberg, branch chief, AFIOH/RSRH Dr. Leo Cropper, Influenza Surveillance Program lead
1000-1100	**Visit to Texas Metro Health**
1130	Lunch
1245-1430	**Site visit to Lackland AFB, tour of the EOS Project** Escorted by: Lt. Col. Sjoberg
1530-1630	**Final review/questions for IOM team/AFIOH** Met by: IOM team Col. Paul Barnicott, deputy commander AFIOH Col. Carolyn Miller, director, SD Lt. Col. Ronald Rippetoe, division chief, AFIOH/SDE Lt. Col. Candace McCall, division chief, AFIOH/RSR Lt. Col. Paul Sjoberg, branch chief, AFIOH/RSRH Dr. Leo Cropper, Influenza Surveillance Program lead Influenza team members

10

Overarching Conclusions and Recommendations

In the preceding chapters the committee has provided site-specific conclusions and recommendations for improving the avian influenza/pandemic influenza (AI/PI) activities of the Department of Defense Global Emerging Infections Surveillance and Response System (DoD-GEIS) at DoD-GEIS headquarters and at each of the DoD-GEIS-supported laboratories. This chapter outlines the committee's overarching recommendations for the DoD-GEIS influenza program and describes the steps the committee feels that the program should take in order to achieve and strengthen a sustained DoD-GEIS influenza surveillance and response effort.

These recommendations are based on the following evaluation criteria identified by DoD-GEIS: (1) consistency with DoD and national plans; (2) the utility of each funded project's contribution to a comprehensive AI/PI surveillance program; (3) adequacy of the program in view of the evolving epidemiologic factors; and (4) coordination of efforts with the Centers for Disease Control and Prevention (CDC), the World Health Organization (WHO), and local governments. In addition, these recommendations seek to address the DoD-GEIS response to the congressional mandate of Sec. 748, H.R.1815, Pandemic Avian Flu Preparedness. Points 7 through 9 from this mandate relate specifically to DoD-GEIS:

(7) Surveillance efforts domestically and internationally, including those using the Global Emerging Infections Systems (GEIS), and how such efforts are integrated with other ongoing surveillance systems.

(8) The integration of pandemic and response planning in the Depart-

ment of Defense with the planning of other Federal departments, including the Department of Health and Human Services, the Department of Homeland Security, the Department of Veterans Affairs, the Department of State, and USAID.

(9) Collaboration (as appropriate) with international entities engaged in pandemic preparedness and response.

CONSISTENCY WITH DEPARTMENT OF DEFENSE AND NATIONAL PLANS

Department of Defense Plans

Executive Agency

Before 1997 the DoD influenza surveillance program consisted largely of the surveillance program of the U.S. Air Force. With the establishment of GEIS in the late 1990s and, more recently, with the $39 million fiscal year 2006 avian influenza supplement, the program has grown to include efforts far beyond those of the historic air force program (see Figure 10-1). These efforts include multimillion-dollar programs at the five DoD overseas labs and at the Naval Health Research Center in San Diego.

Some of these new players have built enough independent laboratory capacity that they no longer are dependent on the laboratory services of the Air Force Institute for Operational Health (AFIOH). This has effectively moved AFIOH toward the margin. This independence from AFIOH and the difficulty that AFIOH experiences in directing and assembling timely data from a myriad of non-air force entities scattered around the world suggests that the overall DoD influenza effort should be administratively reorganized so as to effect better communications, direction, and data management.

RECOMMENDATION 10-1. The executive agency functions of the DoD influenza and respiratory disease surveillance program should be reexamined in light of the evolution of the program in response to the potential of pandemic influenza. DoD-GEIS headquarters should be formally charged with providing managerial and technical oversight (quality assurance, safety, etc.) of the multi-service influenza and respiratory disease program and of the revised structure, including a codified chain of accountability.

A key part of this recommendation would be to tie the funding source (GEIS headquarters) to the global oversight function by moving the executive agency from AFIOH (see Box 9-1) to GEIS headquarters. This tran-

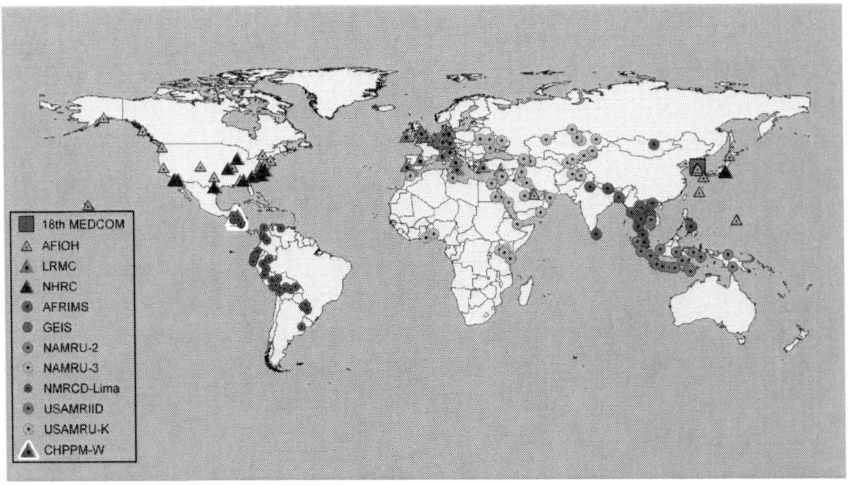

FIGURE 10-1 Department of Defense influenza surveillance sites worldwide, 2007.
SOURCE: DoD-GEIS, 2007b.

sition would strengthen DoD-GEIS headquarters' leadership role in the execution of DoD-GEIS influenza activities as well as improve the execution of the program. Relocating the top-level leadership, data synthesis, and coordination functions to GEIS headquarters makes sense for a number of reasons: GEIS headquarters has growing technical depth with respect to influenza; it is located near the Walter Reed Army Institute of Research and the Naval Medical Research Center headquarters for the DoD overseas labs (which between them are conducting most of the surveillance); it is located near the U.S Food and Drug Administration (FDA); and it is located near most of the key offices for DoD health leadership and influenza leadership at the Department of Health and Human Services (HHS).

DoD Communication and Coordination

The current level of collaboration among domestic and overseas laboratories and between the overseas laboratories and the DoD-GEIS headquarters is commendable, but it could be improved. Despite efforts to foster interlaboratory dialogue and information sharing, certain laboratories appeared to be working in isolation and would benefit from additional information sharing and closer collaboration. Most laboratories are relatively new to the influenza field, and the learning curve over the past fiscal year has been steep.

RECOMMENDATION 10-2. Structured communication mechanisms should be strengthened between DoD-GEIS headquarters and field sites (domestic and international) as well as among sites to create a functional network to enhance coordination of influenza and respiratory disease surveillance activities (epidemiologic, clinical, and laboratory) and to share best practices among all sites.

Each laboratory has learned valuable lessons in using the first year of the supplemental AI/PI funds, and, if shared, these lessons would greatly improve the continued program development of AI/PI activities at all DoD-GEIS sites. Increased interlaboratory dialogue could decrease the likelihood of unintentional overlap of activities between different units and encourage more coordination of activities. Examples of possible mechanisms and tools used for coordination by DoD-GEIS would be monthly teleconferences, periodic website surveillance summaries (with host country concurrence), annual face-to-face meeting—for example, in conjunction with the annual American Society for Tropical Medicine and Hygiene meeting—and sharing of information technologies.

RECOMMENDATION 10-3. In Asia, the Naval Medical Research Unit No. 2 (Indonesia) and the Armed Forces Research Institute of Medical Sciences (Thailand) should work together with DoD-GEIS headquarters to clarify the regional roles of each laboratory and to identify critical geographic areas requiring assistance to strengthen AI/PI surveillance programs in conjunction with World Health Organization and member states regional plans. The laboratories should coordinate the assignment of additional activities as well as prepare contingency plans to cover for each other in the event of a crisis (political, geologic, etc). The same recommendation applies to Africa and the roles of the Naval Medical Research Unit No. 3 (Egypt) and the U.S. Army Medical Research Unit-Kenya. DoD-GEIS headquarters should also work with the Naval Medical Research Center Detachment (Peru) to optimize its regional role in conjunction with Pan American Health Organization and member states regional plans.

National Plans

DoD-GEIS, through its AI/PI activities at the overseas laboratories and headquarters, has contributed greatly to the development of laboratory and communications infrastructures within partner countries. Beneficial effects can be seen from current DoD-GEIS efforts in 56 countries to assist its public health partners in building capacity through training and support of laboratory and communications infrastructures. Within the DoD, GEIS is building capacity directly by supporting the development and maintenance of laboratory diagnostic capacity and indirectly through funding of projects that result in the development of laboratory infrastructure. However, sustaining and expanding DoD laboratory diagnostic capacity is an important activity that could be better and more directly addressed. In their continued implementation of AI/PI projects, GEIS headquarters and laboratories should consider the need to establish sustainable efforts to provide capacity to the host country even if funding is cut. As much as possible, in the selection of equipment and the support of influenza activities, specific items should be purchased that give host-country personnel the best chances of sustainability in meeting their needs within their local setting; when making these choices, the directive to coordinate plans and activities with the host country should be kept in mind.

RECOMMENDATION 10-4. DoD-GEIS funding should be coordinated with funding from all sources to assure the likelihood that surveillance activities for influenza, other respiratory infections, and other emerging infections will be sustainable in overseas sites for the long term.

THE UTILITY OF EACH FUNDED PROJECT'S CONTRIBUTION TO A COMPREHENSIVE AI/PI SURVEILLANCE PROGRAM

While each individual project could not be evaluated in great detail given the available time and resources and the relative infancy of new initiatives,[1] the committee focused on assessing the utility of the DoD laboratories, given their extensive infrastructures and networks for the conduct of infectious studies in the field, to contribute to comprehensive AI/PI surveillance. The DoD units were established at various times between 1942 and 1983, each with a fundamental primary mission of carrying out research relevant to the health of military personnel (DoD-GEIS, 2007a). Over the years, the overseas laboratories have expanded their roles in host countries and in the surrounding geographic regions to include training activities, outbreak responses, and collaborative studies of pathogens of importance to the host nation; but taking on an extensive surveillance role, such as the AI/PI surveillance program, has been a significant departure from their portfolio as it existed prior to the establishment of DoD-GEIS.

The laboratory budgets reflect the current balance of these activities (see Table 10-1). While the fiscal year 2006 AI/PI supplemental funds represent a significant increase in the DoD-GEIS funding going to these laboratories,

[1]Related site-specific committee conclusions and recommendations are included in the appropriate chapters.

TABLE 10-1 Department of Defense Laboratories Funding for Fiscal Year 2006

Organization Funded	DoD-GEIS AI/PI Funding (Thousands)	Other DoD-GEIS Funding (Thousands)	Total Laboratory Funding (Thousands)	Percent of Laboratory Funding Made up by DoD-GEIS
NAMRU-2	$2,665	$1,340	$11,040	36%
AFRIMS	$6,140	$1,340	$18,868	40%
NAMRU-3	$3,988	$1,340	$14,000	38%
USAMRU-K	$2,634	$900	$15,000	24%
NMRCD	$1,741	$1,340	$9,400	33%
NHRC	$3,164	$954	$24,500	17%
AFIOH	$4,182	$713	$42,100	12%
Total	$24,514	$7,927	$134,908	24%

SOURCE: DoD-GEIS and DoD laboratory budget data for fiscal year 2006.

overall DoD-GEIS funds still represent, on average, only 24 percent of the total funding for projects at these DoD laboratories. The majority of the laboratories' funds remain committed to research-oriented projects. It is the committee's view, however, that the surveillance and research activities are complementary to one another. Research contributes to basic scientific knowledge and methods, while the public health surveillance identifies issues that need research and contributes to the overall health and security of host countries and the global community.

The AI/PI surveillance program has built on established relationships and has expanded collaborative activities to include a broader public health agenda. For some overseas laboratories, the implementation of the AI/PI program has been a considerable challenge, with the introduction of a new disease area, new relationships with national and international agencies, and new collaborative opportunities in national and international surveillance activities. In general, though, the overseas laboratories have been successful in developing beneficial ties with appropriate host government components and universities in areas of mutual interest or expertise, with the more established laboratories being particularly successful. Strategic long-term planning for pandemic influenza-preparedness surveillance and response programs, supported by stable funding, would enable the DoD laboratories to determine the appropriate combination of research and public health surveillance needed to best meet the challenge of pandemic influenza as well as other possible emerging pathogens in their areas of responsibility.

RECOMMENDATION 10-5. DoD should issue a directive reaffirming that these traditionally research-oriented laboratories, particularly overseas, have a public health mission with respect to the host country and region; the directive should also provide strategic direction on the balance of military medicine-related research and public health activities.

ADEQUACY OF THE PROGRAM IN VIEW OF EVOLVING EPIDEMIOLOGIC FACTORS

Influenza Surveillance

Using supplemental funding, DoD laboratories have established or improved influenza surveillance in all of their areas of responsibility. With continued funding, both the quality and the utility of surveillance information should improve. The following sections contain recommendations which the committee felt applied to multiple DoD-GEIS surveillance programs. Specific recommendations for each laboratory's activities are in the laboratory-specific chapters.

Human Influenza Surveillance

Institutionalizing influenza surveillance in host countries and within the populations of these host countries provides DoD-GEIS laboratories with opportunities to assist host governments in using the data to prioritize future surveillance activities. Expanding the scope of data collection and analysis to look beyond H5N1 and developing surveillance activities that are amenable to other emerging diseases would greatly benefit overall public health capacity.

Military-to-military partnerships, in which militaries with advanced public health capabilities commit to helping other militaries develop laboratory and epidemiologic capacity, are another way of improving surveillance in developing country militaries (Chretien et al., 2007). Acute respiratory diseases, including viral pathogens such as influenza, have been of special interest to all militaries. The influenza pandemic of 1918 had a devastating impact upon military operations.

There are also methodological advantages for using military populations for influenza surveillance including regimentation of the population, known denominators, and quality of resources for care. An additional benefit of implementing a febrile respiratory infections surveillance and response program through a DoD entity is the strong relationship with the host-country military that DoD-GEIS laboratories can build upon. DoD-GEIS has opportunities to partner with militaries from host countries to improve surveillance capabilities and public health infrastructure (Chretien et al., 2007). DoD-GEIS projects have already found ways to leverage military-to-military relationships to expand surveillance capabilities in both Thailand and Peru (AFRIMS, 2007, NMRCD, 2006).

RECOMMENDATION 10-6. DoD-GEIS programs in the overseas laboratories should explore opportunities to develop or strengthen military influenza surveillance activities in collaboration with host-country military populations.

Animal Influenza Surveillance

Most of the DoD-GEIS laboratories that received AI/PI supplemental funds are implementing animal surveillance programs, a majority of which are in wild bird populations (Table 10-2).

Historically there has been no country in which H5N1 highly pathogenic avian influenza (HPAI) was first detected in healthy wild birds. Prevalence of H5N1 highly pathogenic avian influenza in wild birds has historically been low; therefore sampling numbers need to be sufficiently large to detect the virus. In addition, wild bird surveillance must be appropriately targeted to be of value. Capturing wild birds is difficult, especially migratory wild birds, and, depending on the species, requires expertise and a substantial amount of money. Surveillance should be cost-effective. In most cases, surveillance of mortality events is more fruitful.

Despite the challenges, wild bird surveillance can, if done well, yield useful information on highly pathogenic influenza viruses. Understanding the influenza transmission cycles that involve humans is of value in the areas where labs are located. While the DoD-GEIS strategy of assessing relevant transmission cycles should focus on human testing, teasing out transmission cycles from wild birds to domestic animals to humans is a relevant part of DoD-GEIS influenza research and surveillance projects.

The committee noted that DoD-GEIS could provide valuable expertise at the country level with the integration of animal and human surveillance activities. Better coordination is needed at all levels between human surveillance activities and surveillance for influenza viruses in domestic birds (which have more opportunities to transmit influenza viruses to humans than do free-flying birds) and in other animals. Inadequate coordination affects both the effectiveness of the DoD laboratories and the quality of integrated information regarding the presence of influenza viruses being reported from the host country. DoD-GEIS laboratory personnel could serve

TABLE 10-2 Animal Surveillance Activities at the DoD Overseas Laboratories

DoD Overseas Laboratory	Animal Surveillance Activities
NAMRU-2	NAMRU-2 works with the Indonesian government to develop and conduct surveillance of avian influenza viruses in migratory and wild birds, to train Indonesian government scientists in field and laboratory techniques for collecting and testing for virus, and to use remote sensing to determine environmental correlates for transmission.
AFRIMS	AFRIMS provides laboratory support to the Thai government's animal surveillance activities.
NAMRU-3	NAMRU-3 supports avian influenza surveillance in migratory birds in Ukraine, Egypt, and Kenya with such partners as the Egyptian Ministry of the Environment. In addition, NAMRU-3 acts as a reference laboratory in the EMRO region for other suspected H5N1 animal cases.
USAMRU-K	Working with NAMRU-3, USAMRU-K conducts surveillance to detect highly pathogenic H5 and H7 influenza viruses (or other highly pathogenic influenza viruses) in ducks and other waders as they migrate from Europe and Asia.
NMRCD	NMRCD participates in the Global Avian Influenza Network Surveillance, managed by the World Wildlife Conservation Society at the Bronx Zoo as well as provides veterinary diagnostic support for ongoing Peruvian government activities.

SOURCE: DoD laboratories, DoD-GEIS annual report.

as catalysts to enhance dialogue between national agencies responsible for each of these activities.

RECOMMENDATION 10-7. DoD-GEIS headquarters should assess all of the current wild and domestic bird and animal surveillance activities and firmly establish goals, specifically targeting species and situations to fulfill these goals. DoD-GEIS headquarters and laboratories should seek collaborative opportunities to partner with organizations already studying influenza transmission in wild and domestic birds and animals in their areas.

Laboratory

The AI/PI supplemental funding has been allocated for expanding or enhancing physical structure and laboratory capacity in all of the DoD-GEIS-supported sites (Table 10-3).

TABLE 10-3 Laboratory Capabilities at the DoD Domestic and Overseas Laboratories

	Laboratory Capabilities		
DoD Laboratory	BSL-3	PCR	Multiplex System
NAMRU-2	The construction of BSL-3 at Litbangkes is under way and expected to be completed in 2008.	Yes	Yes
AFRIMS	The design and construction of a BSL-3 lab is under way and expected to be completed by early 2008.	Yes	Yes
NAMRU-3	Yes	Yes	No
USAMRU-K	No[a]	Yes	No
NMRCD	Yes	Yes	No
NHRC	The design and construction of a BSL-3 lab is under way.	Yes	No
AFIOH	Yes	Yes	No

[a]While they do not operate a BSL-3 facility themselves, USAMRU-K and the Kenyan NIC do have access to a BSL-3 laboratory on the grounds of KEMRI.
SOURCE: DoD laboratories, DoD-GEIS annual report.

All of the laboratories have added systems based on reverse transcription polymerase chain reaction (RT-PCR) to increase laboratory throughput and increase their diagnostic capacity. Many of the sites have also used the supplemental funds to increase the biosafety levels of their laboratory space in order to be able to manage highly pathogenic human and animal influenza A viruses. To appropriately staff the laboratories, new personnel with substantial expertise have been hired. All of the improvements to the laboratory facilities have great potential to increase capacity, improve data quality, and ensure rapid identification of the viruses detected.

RECOMMENDATION 10-8. To achieve successful influenza virus surveillance, each of the DoD overseas labs should have the capacity to provide reliable, definitive influenza diagnostic results in a safe and timely way.

Additionally, the expansion of laboratory capacity in domestic and overseas DoD laboratories has the potential to expand each laboratory's autonomy and self-sufficiency in terms of virus isolation and identification as well as in terms of decreasing the reliance on off-site and sometimes distant laboratory facilities. This in-house capacity will also increase the speed at which accurate results are available for decision makers. As the laboratory capacities expand, DoD facilities will need to implement proper procedures to ensure quality assurance.

RECOMMENDATION 10-9. In keeping with the goal of detecting newly recognized drifted or shifted influenza virus (or other emerging pathogens), the DoD-GEIS AI/PI surveillance system should be designed to capture influenza illness that could potentially present with different or unusual symptoms (e.g. conjunctivitis and diarrhea), bringing in outside help and support in the case of novel findings.

Response Capacity

The period between the first convincing evidence of human-to-human transmission of a pandemic strain in one or more geographic areas and the subsequent widespread transmission of the disease worldwide could range from a few weeks to a few months. During that period laboratory testing can determine where the pandemic strain is and where it is not. Once the first clusters of human–to-human transmission have been unequivocally identified, any outbreak of respiratory illness anywhere in the world will likely create concern (and even panic) that the illness is caused by the emerging pandemic virus. Ruling out a pandemic strain as being responsible for influenza-like illness in a community could avoid or lessen panic and confusion among the general population. Rapid testing may help limit overreactions and reduce needless depletion of antivirals, vaccines, masks, and other protective stocks.

Laboratories must be prepared for expanded laboratory-based surveillance activities during this critical period between the initial epidemiologic harbingers of an influenza pandemic and eventual global spread. Laboratories currently testing a few samples a day, a week, or a month will be called upon to test many more during this period. Without necessarily adding new instruments or expanding in space, these laboratories could gear up to work more shifts if they could deploy trained lab technicians from other parts of the lab and rely upon sufficient supplies of reagents to perform the tests. Taking the steps of redeploying technicians and working in shifts would be facilitated if a lab has already devised a surge capacity plan, trained the other lab staff, and secured a source of reagents and supplies. Developing a surge capacity plan prior to human-to-human transmission could mean

TABLE 10-4 Estimated Laboratory Surge Capacity at DoD Domestic and Overseas Laboratories

Laboratory	Routine Operation	Altered Algorithm (Flu A & H5 first)	Target H5 Gene Only	24-Hours–a-Day, Seven-Days-a-Week Operations
NAMRU-2	360/week	4,900/week	11,000/week	19,200/week
AFRIMS	400/week	600/week	2,000/week	5,000/week
NAMRU-3	2,250/week	3,400/week	***	8,800/week
USAMRU-K	200/week	2,000/week	2,000/week	4,000/week
NMRCD	300/week	***	***	1,300/week
NHRC	336/week	1,112/week	1,988/week	4,760/week
AFIOH	1,300 /week	***	1,500/week	6,000/week

SOURCE: DoD laboratories surge capacity estimates.

adapting to the increase in the number of samples in a few hours instead of days or weeks.

Each of the DoD domestic and overseas laboratories estimated its own surge capacity in the event of an influenza pandemic in its host country (Table 10-4). The committee found that surge planning within these laboratories as well as the strategic planning at the DoD-GEIS headquarters level could be greatly strengthened. The inadequacies of the central DoD-GEIS strategy with respect to the role of laboratories' surge capacities in their areas of responsibility, especially in the case of a pandemic, will leave the laboratories unprepared in the efforts to best assist host governments and multilateral partners.

While it is useful to understand how the DoD laboratories could contribute in a pandemic, in many countries there are no estimates of needed laboratory surge capacity with which to put the DoD laboratories' contribution into context. In the event of a pandemic, the DoD laboratory network will serve as only one piece of the required surge capacity, and at the current time it is unclear what role each laboratory will play.

RECOMMENDATION 10-10. The DoD-GEIS influenza surveillance programs in the overseas laboratories should be complementary to the host-country laboratory system and help to increase surge capacity at the host country levels. DoD-GEIS should work with CDC, WHO, the U.S. Department of Agriculture, the Food and Agricultural Organiza-

tion, and other entities at the headquarters and in-country levels to develop a plan to handle an increased number of influenza samples from humans or animals.

Information Sharing

An effective surveillance network detects cases of disease, collects and analyzes the data, and disseminates the findings to people and organizations that use the information. For influenza, rapid and effective communication of information is essential for public health partners positioned to respond, such as ministries of health, U.S. partner agencies, and international organizations. Strategies for sharing information with public health partners have not been formally developed, although in most laboratories good practices have evolved.

Methods and needs for sharing data vary greatly within the DoD-GEIS consortium, but information needs must be assessed and communication channels identified and opened. Equally important are the needs for the DoD-GEIS headquarters to collect surveillance data and other information from consortium members in a systematic, timely manner, analyze this information as appropriate, and report this information back to consortium members and other relevant DoD personnel, public health partners, and the public. Each of the domestic and overseas laboratories has developed slightly different methods of sharing results among stakeholders (Table 10-5).

Current DoD-GEIS efforts to communicate influenza virus surveillance and other information within the DoD-GEIS consortium, within the DoD, to public health partners, and to the public are improving but remain insufficient. Of particular concern is the need for effective communication and dissemination of results as well as isolates at both the executive-agent and in-country levels. There must be a clear understanding of how and when information and specimens are to be communicated from the laboratories to WHO through the host country government and to the U.S. public health system via DoD. There is an established international system organized by WHO for flow of information and of influenza virus isolates from humans and animals. It was unclear in some places how DoD-GEIS laboratories were working with host governments to ensure that information was being fed into the WHO system. The channels of information flow from DoD-GEIS-supported activities and isolate distribution must be clearly understood by the host country and relevant international organizations.

RECOMMENDATION 10-11. DoD-GEIS influenza surveillance programs in the overseas laboratories in each host country should have a written understanding among all national and international partners

delineating the reporting of influenza virus detections and the appropriate channels for exchanging isolates and communicating virological results. Such a document should include a clear statement of the laboratory designated by WHO as the reference laboratory for isolates from the host country.

COORDINATION OF EFFORTS WITH THE CENTERS FOR DISEASE CONTROL AND PREVENTION, THE WORLD HEALTH ORGANIZATION, AND LOCAL GOVERNMENTS

Addressing emerging infectious diseases is an issue of global importance and shared responsibility. It is crucial to the success of a global influenza surveillance system that all of the relevant partners work together to plan and prepare for a possible pandemic. To this end, DoD-GEIS is working to

TABLE 10-5 Information Sharing at DoD Domestic and Overseas Laboratories

DoD Laboratory	Description of Laboratory Data Sharing Practices
NAMRU-2	Isolates are sent from NAMRU-2 to the Indonesian Ministry of Health and subsequently to CDC-Atlanta for analysis as part of its annual influenza vaccine development activities.
AFRIMS	Isolates are provided from AFRIMS to the Thai Ministry of Public Health according to Thai regulations and for subsequent reporting to the WHO.
NAMRU-3	All isolates are forwarded to the CDC and/or Mill Hill (United Kingdom) as WHO collaborating centers. Results are reported to the Ministry of Health, WHO, and NAMRU-3 or other influenza partners as appropriate (i.e., DoD-GEIS, NMRC, CDC, etc.).
USAMRU-K	Isolates are provided from USAMRU-K to the Kenya Medical Research Institute.
NMRCD	Monthly reporting to the Ministry of Health, participating physicians, and the Air Force Institute for Operational Health in San Antonio, Texas.
NHRC	NHRC sends out a weekly newsletter that updates influenza activity seen in all its surveillance programs to many DoD stakeholders. Influenza viral sequence information is reported to the CDC.
AFIOH	AFIOH provides select isolates and all sequence data to the CDC and WHO for further subtyping and antigenic characterization for detection of variance from the vaccine component strains.

SOURCE: DoD laboratories, DoD-GEIS annual report.

coordinate and integrate its efforts with national and international surveillance and response-planning partners, such as CDC, HHS, the Pan American Health Organization (PAHO), WHO, and the U.S. Department of Agriculture's Animal and Plant Health Inspection Service. At the time of the site visits, DoD-GEIS surveillance activities were integrated with those of U.S. government, host country, and multilateral partners to various degrees often dependent on how long each program had been underway. However, DoD-GEIS headquarters and all of the domestic and overseas laboratories were working to improve the levels of coordination and integration using AI/PI supplemental funds.

International Partners

Congress, as expressed in Sec. 748, H.R.1815, and the DoD strategic plan both call for DoD-GEIS to collaborate with international partners, such as WHO, and with governmental agencies in foreign countries, such as ministries of health. With the supplemental funding, DoD-GEIS has been working on expanding its influenza activities in coordination with international partners. At the headquarters level, the assignment of a full-time U.S. military medical officer to WHO in Geneva, Switzerland, has bolstered coordination and integration of efforts between DoD-GEIS and WHO (Fukuda, 2006). In addition, DoD-GEIS seeks external advice and consultation for AI/PI surveillance and control activities on a project-by-project basis from outside consultants, such as key offices at PAHO, WHO, and the Food and Agricultural Organization, as needed.

DoD-GEIS has 260 influenza surveillance sites in 56 countries around the world (see Figure 10-2). A number of these countries represent collaborations with WHO national influenza centers and other international partners.

The DoD laboratories also play a significant role in the establishment of collaborative relationships with international partners and governmental agencies in foreign countries. At a number of DoD laboratories the implementation of the supplemental funding has lead to the strengthening of these relationships. The DoD overseas laboratories have developed and significantly improved relationships with a variety of global and host-country partners working in the fields of avian and pandemic influenza (see Table 10-6).

In addition, a number of the DoD overseas laboratories have increased international collaboration and coordination by serving dual functions as U.S. DoD laboratories as well as WHO collaborating centers or reference laboratories (Table 10-7).

While significant effort has been put into strengthening the coordination of avian and pandemic influenza activities, the overseas laboratories

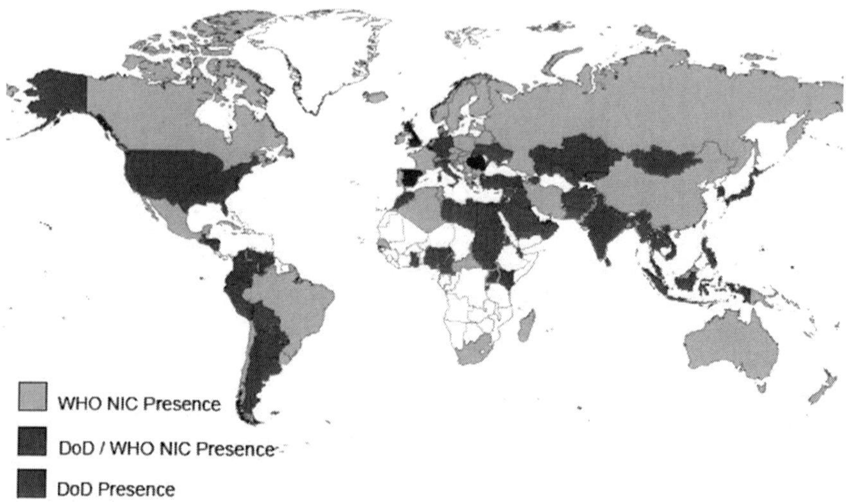

FIGURE 10-2 DoD's worldwide presence in influenza surveillance, 2007.
SOURCE: DoD-GEIS, 2006.

TABLE 10-6 International Partners of DoD Overseas Laboratories

DoD Laboratory	Global and Host-Country Partners
NAMRU-2	Indonesian Ministry of Health, Indonesian Ministry of Agriculture and Fisheries, Indonesian National Institutes of Health Research and Development (Litbangkes), WHO, FAO, other partner governments in the region
AFRIMS	Royal Thai Army, Thailand Ministry of Public Health, Thai Ministry of Agriculture and Cooperatives, WHO, other partner governments in the region
NAMRU-3	Egyptian ministries of health, environment, and agriculture, WHO EMRO, FAO, APHIS, other partner governments in the region
USAMRU-K	Kenya Medical Research Institute (KEMRI), AFIOH, and Kenya Ministry of Health (KMoH) Ministry of Livestock and Fisheries, ornithology department of the National Museums of Kenya, Kenya Wildlife Service, WHO, GTZ, FAO, other partner governments in the region
NMRCD	Peruvian Ministry of Health, Ministry of Agriculture, and Military, PAHO, other partner governments in the region

SOURCE: DoD laboratories, DoD-GEIS annual report.

TABLE 10-7 DoD Laboratories Serving as WHO Collaborating Centers and Reference Laboratories

DoD Laboratory	WHO Role
NAMRU-2	WHO Collaborating Centre for New, Emerging and Reemerging Infectious Diseases
AFRIMS	WHO Collaborating Center for Diagnostic Reference, Training, and Investigation of Emerging Infectious Diseases
NAMRU-3	WHO Regional Influenza Reference Laboratory and WHO reference laboratories for diagnosis of influenza A/H5 infection

SOURCE: DoD laboratories, DoD-GEIS annual report.

must continue their efforts to work within each country's national plan, thereby increasing national capacity and avoiding unintentionally working against the national plan. DoD influenza protocols should be executed in such a way that they cause a net strengthening of national and international capacity. As part of these collaborations, the overseas laboratories should also take opportunities to assist the host country in the development and implementation of disease-control guidelines and pandemic preparedness where appropriate and necessary. In some countries, for example, the committee found a lack of evidence of influenza pandemic preparedness at the local hospital level.

RECOMMENDATION 10-12. Overseas laboratories, with the strategic guidance of DoD-GEIS headquarters, should coordinate with national and regional influenza pandemic and enzootic response plans to establish the role for each laboratory in country and regionally. Where possible, DoD-GEIS laboratories should engage in host-country influenza coordinating activities, including tabletop response exercises and distribution of testing capacity, in concert with WHO and other international agencies. An important goal will be to strengthen linkages between laboratories and entities with key resources.

U.S. Government Partners

The DoD is also one of several U.S. government agencies with a significant interest in and responsibility for addressing emerging infectious diseases such as influenza. Each agency fills a particular niche and contributes important resources while also having certain limitations. The DoD, for its part, possesses unique laboratory capabilities, many situated in diverse forward locations, and has a vested interest in addressing emerging infectious diseases as a matter of national security (NIC, 2000).

While the DoD will have limited public health role in the event of a pandemic in the U.S. according to the National Strategy for Pandemic Influenza, Implementation Plan (see Box 10-1), the influenza surveillance activities being conducted at the DoD's domestic and overseas laboratories are producing valuable information on the location and variations of the circulating influenza viruses which can help prepare both U.S. military and civilian populations.

In order to ensure coordinated U.S. government planning and implementation of influenza activities, DoD-GEIS-supported personnel work to coordinate influenza-related activities with other U.S. government agencies both at headquarters and at the laboratory level. At the headquarters level, DoD-GEIS staff participates in a number of influenza-coordinating

BOX 10-1
National Strategy for Pandemic Influenza, Implementation Plan Roles and Responsibilities

The **Secretary of Homeland Security** will be responsible for coordination of the federal response as provided by the National Strategy for Pandemic Influenza (Strategy), and will support the Secretary of Health and Human Services' coordination of overall public health and medical emergency response efforts.

The **Secretary of Health and Human Services** will be responsible for the overall coordination of the public health and medical emergency response during a pandemic.

The **Secretary of Defense** will be responsible for protecting American interests at home and abroad.

The **Secretary of Transportation** will be responsible for coordination of the transportation sector.

The **Secretary of Agriculture** will be responsible for overall coordination of veterinary response to a domestic animal outbreak of a pandemic virus or virus with pandemic potential and ongoing surveillance for influenza in domestic animals and animal products.

The **Secretary of the Treasury** will be responsible for monitoring and evaluating the economic impacts of the pandemic and will help formulate the economic policy response and advise on the likely economic impacts of containment efforts.

Other cabinet heads will retain responsibility for their respective sectors and will be responsible for developing pandemic.

bodies, including annual DoD Joint Influenza Surveillance Working Group meetings as well as a number of HHS-coordinated influenza-related groups (Embrey, 2006). DoD representatives also participate with other U.S. government partners at the annual meetings of the FDA-sponsored Vaccines and Related Biological Products Advisory Committee. DoD and other government agencies, including HHS, the Department of Homeland Security, the State Department, and CDC, have exchanged full-time medical liaison officers to help provide situational awareness of ongoing missions and to implement initiatives of mutual interest (Bresee and Jernigan, 2006).

DoD domestic and overseas laboratories have been working to improve their collaborations with other relevant U.S. agencies working in the same locations, including other DoD entities, CDC, the U.S. Agency for International Development (USAID), the U.S. Department of Agriculture (USDA), and the National Aeronautics and Space Administration. (See Table 10-8 for a list of DoD laboratories and their U.S. government partners.) The roles of various DoD laboratories in the event of a pandemic are less clear in the host country setting. The responsibilities of each U.S. government agency should be agreed upon by each U.S. agency and outlined by the host country government.

The relationship between the CDC and the DoD warrants particular attention. The CDC now has a presence in almost all of the countries where the overseas laboratories are located. In the past the DoD and the CDC have provided each other with backup support and entered into collaborative relationships on an as-needed basis. As influenza activities evolve, collaboration between the CDC and the DoD will be of utmost importance if

TABLE 10-8 U.S. Government Partners of DoD Domestic and Overseas Laboratories

DoD Laboratory	US Agency Partners
NAMRU-2	CDC, USAID, NASA, U.S. Embassy, AFRIMS
AFRIMS	CDC, USAID, NAMRU-2, AFIOH
NAMRU-3	CDC, USAID
USAMRU-K	CDC, USAID, AFIOH, NAMRU-3
NMRCD	CDC, USAID, AFIOH, USDA
NHRC	CDC, AFIOH, NAMRU-2, NAMRU-3, USDA
AFIOH	CDC, AFRIMS, USAMRU-K, NMRCD, NHRC, USCHPPM,

SOURCE: DoD laboratories, DoD-GEIS annual report.

both are to make efficient and effective use of limited resources. Similarly, strong relationships with other U.S. government partners such as USAID and USDA ensure most efficient use of U.S. funds.

RECOMMENDATION 10-13. DoD-GEIS should further strengthen its coordination and collaboration on pandemic influenza and other emerging infectious diseases with all U.S. partners, both domestically and in its overseas operations. These partners include HHS, CDC, the National Institutes of Health, FDA, USDA, the Department of State, the U.S. Agency for International Development, the Department of Homeland Security, and other relevant U.S. government efforts.

CONCLUSION

Overall, the committee concluded that DoD-GEIS has effectively executed and managed the fiscal year 2006 AI/PI supplemental funding, especially given condensed timeframes for planning and implementation. At DoD-GEIS headquarters, as well as at the domestic and overseas laboratories, DoD-GEIS personnel absorbed the increase in funding into programs aimed at successfully building DoD and host-country laboratory and human resource capacity, globally expanding information about avian influenza and acute respiratory diseases, benefitting the health of U.S. military personnel, and strengthening U.S. relations within the global community. The preceding sections describe the steps the committee feels that the program should take in order to achieve and strengthen a sustained DoD-GEIS influenza surveillance and response effort. With sustained funding and the implementation of these recommendations, DoD-GEIS has a unique opportunity to further contribute to the evolving global knowledge of highly pathogenic avian influenza virus as well as continue to strengthen global emerging infectious disease surveillance and response.

REFERENCES

AFRIMS (Armed Forces Research Institute of Medical Sciences). 2007. *AFRIMS influenza surveillance program—current and future* (unpublished).

Bresee, J., and D. Jernigan. 2006. *U.S. government contributions to global influenza surveillance*. PowerPoint presentation given at first meeting of the IOM Committee for the Assessment of DoD-GEIS Influenza Surveillance and Response Programs, December 19, Washington, DC.

Chretien, J. P., D. L. Blazes, R. L. Coldren, M. D. Lewis, J. Gaywee, K. Kana, N. Sirisopana, V. Vallejos, C. C. Mundaca, S. Montano, G. J. Martin, and J. C. Gaydos. 2007. The importance of militaries from developing countries in global infectious disease surveillance. *Bulletin of the World Health Organization* 85(3):174-180.

DoD-GEIS (Department of Defense Global Emerging Infections System). 2006. *DoD Global Emerging Infections Surveillance and Response System annual report fiscal year 2006.* Silver Spring, MD: Walter Reed Army Institute for Research

DoD-GEIS. 2007a. *DoD-GEIS website.* http://www.geis.fhp.osd.mil/ (accessed August 7, 2007).

DoD-GEIS. 2007b. *Department of Defense influenza surveillance sites worldwide, 2007* (unpublished).

Embrey, E. P. 2006. *U.S. government policy perspectives on global influenza.* PowerPoint presentation given at first meeting of the IOM Committee for the Assessment of DoD-GEIS Influenza Surveillance and Response Programs, December 19, Washington, DC.

Fukuda, K. 2006. *Global challenges of pandemic and avian influenza.* PowerPoint presentation given at first meeting of the IOM Committee for the Assessment of DoD-GEIS Influenza Surveillance and Response Programs, December 19, Washington, DC.

NIC (National Intelligence Council). 2000. *The global infectious disease threat and its implications for the U.S.* http://www.fas.org/irp/threat/nie99-17d.htm (accessed July 24, 2007).

NMRCD (U.S. Naval Medical Research Center Detachment). 2006. *Influenza and disease surveillance summary* (unpublished).

Appendix

Cumulative Number of Confirmed Human Cases of Avian Influenza A/(H5N1) Reported to WHO, 11 July 2007

	2003		2004		2005		2006		2007		Total	
Country	cases	deaths	cases	deaths	cases	deaths	cases	deaths	cases	deaths	cases	deaths
Azerbaijan	0	0	0	0	0	0	8	5	0	0	8	5
Cambodia	0	0	0	0	4	4	2	2	1	1	7	7
China	1	1	0	0	8	5	13	8	3	2	25	16
Djibouti	0	0	0	0	0	0	1	0	0	0	1	0
Egypt	0	0	0	0	0	0	18	10	19	5	37	15
Indonesia	0	0	0	0	20	13	55	45	27	23	102	81
Iraq	0	0	0	0	0	0	3	2	0	0	3	2
Lao People's Democratic Republic	0	0	0	0	0	0	0	0	2	2	2	2
Nigeria	0	0	0	0	0	0	0	0	1	1	1	1
Thailand	0	0	17	12	5	2	3	3	0	0	25	17
Turkey	0	0	0	0	0	0	12	4	0	0	12	4
Viet Nam	3	3	29	20	61	19	0	0	2	0	95	42
Total	4	4	46	32	98	43	115	79	55	34	318	192

NOTES: Total number of cases includes number of deaths.
WHO reports only laboratory-confirmed cases.
All dates refer to onset of illness.
SOURCE: WHO. 2007. This information was reprinted with permission from WHO.[1]

[1]WHO. 2007. *Cumulative number of confirmed human cases of avian influenza A/(H5N1) reported to WHO*. http://www.who.int/csr/disease/avian_influenza/country/cases_table_2007_07_25/en/index.html (accessed July 27, 2007).